ALSO BY JEAN ANTONELLO

How to Become Naturally Thin by Eating More

JEAN ANTONELLO, R.N., B.S.N.

A FIRESIDE BOOK

PUBLISHED BY SIMON & SCHUSTER

NEW YORK LONDON TORONTO SYDNEY TOKYO SINGAPORE

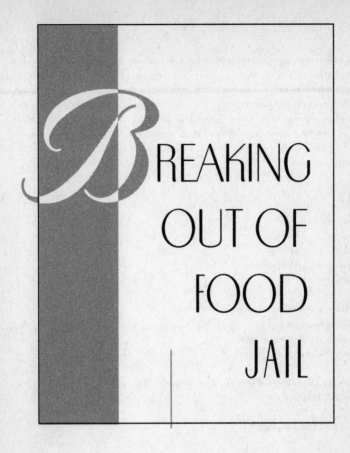

BREAKING OUT OF FOOD JAIL

How to Free Yourself
from Diets
and Problem Eating,
Once and for All

THE RECOMMENDATIONS FOR COPING WITH THE SYMPTOMS OF EATING PROBLEMS IN THIS BOOK
ARE NOT MEANT TO REPLACE MEDICAL THERAPIES. IF YOU ARE UNSURE ABOUT WHETHER YOU ARE
IN ANY PHYSICAL DANGER FROM YOUR DESTRUCTIVE EATING PATTERNS, SEE A HEALTH PROFES-
SIONAL FOR AN EXAMINATION. DO NOT TRY TO TREAT YOURSELF WITHOUT THE APPROVAL OF
YOUR DOCTOR IF YOU ARE UNDER A PHYSICIAN'S CARE. IF ANY OF YOUR SYMPTOMS INDICATE
THAT YOU MAY BE CAUSING HARM TO YOUR BODY, GET MEDICAL HELP. EATING DISTURBANCES
CAN BE HEALTH AND EVEN LIFE THREATENING, MAINLY BECAUSE VICTIMS DENY THE SERIOUSNESS
OF THEIR SYMPTOMS.

FIRESIDE
ROCKEFELLER CENTER
1230 AVENUE OF THE AMERICAS
NEW YORK, NY 10020

DESIGNED BY KAROLINA HARRIS

MANUFACTURED IN THE UNITED STATES OF AMERICA

10 9 8 7 6 5 4 3 2 1

LIBRARY OF CONGRESS CATALOGING-IN-PUBLICATION DATA
ANTONELLO, JEAN.
BREAKING OUT OF FOOD JAIL: HOW TO FREE YOURSELF FROM DIETS
AND PROBLEM EATING ONCE AND FOR ALL/JEAN ANTONELLO.
P.   CM.
INCLUDES INDEX.
1. EATING DISORDERS—PSYCHOLOGICAL ASPECTS. 2. WOMEN—PSYCHOLOGY.
I. TITLE.
RC552.025A56 1996
616.85'26—DC20 —DC20
[616.85'26]   96-820
                    CIP

ISBN 0-684-81193-6

CONTENTS

INTRODUCTION

Statistics do not tell the real stories behind the multitudes of people, especially women and young girls, who suffer chronically from eating problems. You are probably one of them. You feel as if you are at war with your body. Its urges are frightening and uncontrollable at times. You've tried countless vows, rules, tricks and gimmicks to bring your eating behavior under control. And sometimes you've succeeded, for a while. But the price is so high—constant vigilance, preoccupation with food and weight, cravings, fear of losing control—losing control. How did you ever get to this unhappy place? Somehow, it seems, you just woke up in jail—food jail.

The fact is, the path to food jail is well worn and not nearly as mysterious as it appears. There is a definite route to this prison, and just as surely, there is a very real way out—to eating freedom. This path is waiting for you, if you decide to break out. But you will need faith and courage, and the determination to break free.

Eating problems come with all sorts of labels, including compulsive eating, emotional overeating, food addiction, bulimia and anorexia. Often these terms are too strong or rigid to accurately define a person's problem because most struggles with eating behavior are more subtle than true eating disorders. It doesn't really matter, though, because almost *all* troubled eating springs from the same source, and that source is physical, not psychological. With rare exception, eating difficulties arise from the conflict between a person who is trying to restrict food intake and her/his body's survival instinct. This is the foundation of the program detailed in *Breaking Out of Food Jail*.

But wait a minute! Aren't eating disorders rare psychological problems that cannot be cured? Aren't they like drug addictions? Don't people with eating disorders have to get into a program like Alcoholics Anonymous and stick with it for the rest of their lives? Don't they need deep psychotherapy? Aren't some people just born with eating problems so that they can never be rational about food, no matter what? What can possibly be done to help those of us who wrestle with eating demons that isn't being done?

The answers to these questions, which I address in this book, are no, no, no, no, no and A LOT. As an obesity and eating disorders specialist for eight years, I have talked with hundreds who are caught in the trap of what I call disturbed eating. You're in the trap if you have to think about eating or food too much, if it interferes with your life in any way, if it feels unnatural, fearful, extreme or upsetting. You're nodding your head—you've got the right book.

I became determined to write about eating disturbances mainly because of the rampant and destructive prejudices that exist about them. First of all, they are not rare, although they are rarely diagnosed by professionals because distorted eating is always accompanied by shame and guilt, and few who suffer from these problems, even those with serious eating disorders, ever seek help. Most are unaware of the extent of their symptoms or the damage they may be inflicting on their bodies. Denial and secrecy play big roles in eating struggles. Many flatly deny that there is anything unusual about their eating patterns, even though they may be in great psychological and even physical pain. Often they feel fearful and hopeless about getting help, even if they admit that eating is a problem for them.

Although, traditionally, eating disorders have been viewed as psychological problems, I know that these disorders have a powerful *physical* basis. I am convinced that most of the symptoms of these disorders are physical and psychological manifestations of the body's adaptive responses to *undereating behavior*—consciously limiting food intake below your needs. Undereating certainly may have some psychological components, but I have found the culturally induced fear of weight gain to be the single most compelling and universal element, regardless of personal problems or psychological issues. This fact remains: the physical cause of eating disorders has been pretty much ignored until now, and I believe this aspect of modern eating problems is the key to effective and lasting treatment.

The goals of treatment I outlined in this book are:

1. to enjoy a normal relationship with food;
2. to maintain a healthy, lean body weight without anxiety or inordinate effort; and
3. to develop a normal body image.

Sound like your wish list?

I have witnessed complete recoveries of individuals I coached who had suffered from debilitating eating disturbances for years. Many more people said that reading my first book, *How to Become Naturally Thin by Eating More,* helped cure them of seriously disturbed eating patterns. I myself have recovered from years of disturbed eating patterns, so I know that eating problems, even serious ones, can be cured, and I know that being cured is like getting out of jail.

The key to unlocking the mysteries of disturbed eating behavior lies in exposing the cause behind these problems. Effective treatment, which depends on an accurate understanding of eating disturbances, has eluded professionals using the traditional psychological model. *Breaking Out of Food Jail* presents a major departure from this conventional perspective on eating problems by targeting physical cause and physical treatment. Physical treatment guidelines are infinitely simpler, more universal and less time consuming than psychological therapies. Moreover, they are effective where psychological treatments have not been.

Although you may be ready to read this book, you may not be ready to work on your eating problem right now and do the specific exercises designed to move you toward healthier eating patterns. If you are not, relax. You can still read the book, just taking in the information without forcing a premature breakout from food jail. But if you feel you are ready to follow the suggestions in the book, push yourself gently along, remembering to pace, rest and review, with your own special needs in mind.

So much of the last two-thirds of the book hinges on the first third that I recommend reading it straight through, even if you are primarily interested in, say, the chapter on preventing eating problems in kids. This book will completely overhaul your thinking and prejudices about eating problems, and it could be a bit confusing if you put the cart ahead of the horse.

Please mark up the book (if it is yours), highlighting the principles or case studies that are most helpful to you. Dog-ear pages you need to reread, then reread them. Photocopy illustrations, definitions or information that you need to program into your thinking. Hang them on your mirror or over your kitchen sink and review them until they become second nature to you.

Sound drastic? Not when you consider how you ended up in food jail in the first place. You've been in a cult of sorts—call it the diet cult, or anti-eating cult if you like. You are now your own deprogrammer, and this book is the new program designed to get you back in touch with reality about eating, about food, about your body. So don't be timid; your liberation is at stake.

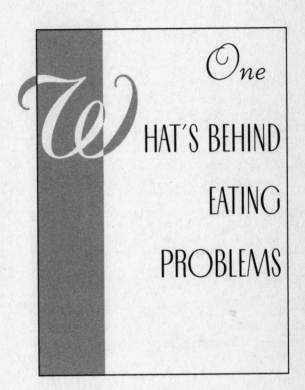

One

WHAT'S BEHIND EATING PROBLEMS

CHAPTER 1

To Eat or Not to Eat, That Is the Obsession

NOWADAYS, THE PERSON WHO IS ABLE TO EAT freely and enjoy her dining experiences from day to day, unhampered by guilt, anxiety and a dozen other pressures, is truly an exception. If you ever come across a person like this, don't you *hate* her? Almost everyone is, at the very least it seems, watching her weight. Most of us have lost our love of food and eating. It has been contaminated by guilts, superstitions, prejudices, false information, undocumented beliefs, crazy body-image standards, fashion pressures, diet madness, excessive and contradictory research studies, and, especially, fear. We are afraid of food. We believe it makes people fat and that, if we don't stay on guard, it will make us fat, too (if we aren't already so, to some degree).

We are, almost as a nation, obsessed with eating less! The calorie is synonymous with evil, and fat grams have come to represent the very measure of success or failure in foods—an inverse relationship, of course. Terms like "low-fat," "low-calorie," "light" or "lean" are an integral part of our vocabularies. We think, talk and read these terms and concepts, meditating on their meaning and influence on our bodies. Eat light, eat less, eat low-fat, we say, if we're among the "liberals" who condone eating at all. We are obsessed this way because we are all afraid of getting fat and we are all positive that too much food, by itself, makes people fat.

But where's all this food avoidance, fat phobia and calorie obsession leading, anyway? For a growing number of people, straight to eating problems.

By the time she was forty-three, Paula had dieted, one way or another, for twenty-five years. In that time she had joined Weight Watchers over ten times, tried Jenny Craig, gave Weight Loss Center two efforts and Optifast just one (because it was so expensive), and attended seven years of regular Overeaters Anonymous meetings. In addition, she had read dozens of books and magazine articles in her attempts to control her eating.

Paula was an expert on nutrition. She knew so much about food groups, calories and fat grams that she could have started her own consulting business, Diet Madness, Inc. She knew by heart and in her sleep what she should eat, exactly how much and when, according to the experts. Paula was queen of portion control and truly gifted at policing fat grams. She had been trying to eat less, eat light, eat low-fat all her adult life. And she had been losing control of her eating for just about as long. Paula couldn't remember back to a time when she wasn't preoccupied with her eating and her weight. Over the years she learned multitudes of diet skills and tips, hints and tricks. And now Paula was heavier and more desperate than she had ever been in her life.

Let's not forget the "enlightened" wave of the nineties: diets don't work in the long run so exercise is the answer! And since most people today have passed through the anti-eating culture of the seventies and eighties, many are adding exercise to their deeply ingrained habits of avoiding food. Work that body fat, jog that belly off, burn that blubber with aerobics! And where are all these underfed, overworked bodies headed? Once again, more and more are headed toward disturbed eating patterns and straight into "food jail."

Just after she turned thirty, Arlene started working out with her boyfriend, who was an avid weight lifter. After they broke up she discovered she had learned to love exercise. At first she just felt sort of a natural high when she finished her aerobics class, but later Arlene noticed that her stomach was getting flatter. That was a plus she hadn't expected. Not long after she was "single" again, one of the personal trainers embarrassed her by making a friendly comment about how great she looked. Arlene was flattered. No one had ever really

*noticed her in this way before. Why not help the process along
with a little dieting? she thought. So the fruit and salads began to replace the sandwiches and pasta.*

*The Friday night of the first week into her new diet/exercise
program, Arlene thought about ice cream as she watched TV.
She had never been into sweets much, so this was unusual for
her. Oh, just a little. I've been so good, she rationalized.*

*Thirty minutes and a quart of Rocky Road later, Arlene
was surprised and a little afraid. A quart of ice cream! What
happened? At first she felt confused, but quickly shifted her
attitude to determination. Tomorrow I'll work out two hours
and just have juice for breakfast, she promised. And she did.
Nothing but a Caesar salad for lunch and plenty of mineral
water to keep the hunger under control. But after a dinner of
broiled fish that night at a restaurant she found herself eating the leftover fries from her friends' plates and drinking
four beers. French fries were definitely forbidden for Arlene.
And beer, well, one was usually enough. Under the influence
of the beer, and her nagging hunger, Arlene topped it all off
with a big fudge brownie delight, complete with ice cream
and hot fudge.*

*Arlene looked at herself in the mirror in the ladies' room at
the restaurant and felt disgusted. What is wrong with me,
anyway? she wondered. I've got to get rid of this feeling—I'm
completely stuffed. I can't stand feeling this full. I'll just throw
up this once, then get back in control. My college roommate
did it all the time and it never hurt her.*

Of course, if we are already fat, we've proven it to ourselves repeatedly: food and lack of exercise have made us fat. We stand as
a warning to others: Beware! This will happen to you, too, if you
eat too much and/or drop your aerobics class. Those who are already overweight are sometimes the most afraid of eating because
they stand as a nonstop warning to themselves: The pounds and
bulges will keep piling on if you don't stop eating so much. Eat
less! Don't eat at all if you can help it! You're not that hungry. Get
some exercise. What's the matter with you?

Is there another way? Is there hope? Is it possible for us to be-
friend food without getting fat? Is there a way to improve our diets
without going off the deep end? Can we ever get back to enjoying
the natural, lifelong pleasure of eating? Can exercise ever be en-

joyable, free of obsessive pressures and fears? And the most important question of all: Can we learn to enjoy eating plenty of good food, have moderate activity levels and be thin, too?

To all of these queries, I answer a resounding YES! Keep reading. The "hows" are just ahead.

THE WRONG TREE

At the heart of all this confusion about food, weight gain and eating struggles lies a very real problem—prejudice, even among professionals and researchers, about the cause of overweight and eating disorders.

For decades we have been taught that overeating and underexercise cause overweight, and that psychological problems cause eating disorders. I believe these two presumptions are overly simplistic and incorrect, and account for the immense frustration within this field of study and among the millions of people who suffer from eating and weight problems. We have truly been barking up the wrong tree in this important field of human behavior, with extremely serious consequences to both mental and physical health for millions of us.

Complete with plenty of diet advertisements, and occasionally an ad for an eating disorders treatment facility, popular women's magazines rarely fail to highlight a weight-loss method on the cover or tell some celebrity's story of weight loss, weight gain or eating disorder. These topics ensure sales because editors know what women are obsessed with. We seem to have an insatiable appetite for information about dieting, weight loss and eating problems, but what we're being fed is almost all junk food.

Everyone in this culture has been programmed by the media and especially by health professionals (who inform the media) to believe that fat people need to eat less and exercise more, and people with eating problems need to see a therapist. Moms and dads learn it from newspaper articles and doctors, and pass it on to their children. Teachers teach it, preachers preach it. There isn't a shadow of a doubt about these two sacred tenets in most people's minds, especially in those who are overweight or eating disturbed themselves. (The term "eating disturbed" applies to anyone for whom eating has become a problem.) The funny thing is, these well-established approaches rarely lead to cures. They cause a lot of people to work hard and dole out plenty of money off and on over decades, but they just never manage to correct the problems they're designed to remedy. In fact, they often make them worse! The reason is simple: The theories behind these treatment methods are not completely true, so the methods cannot succeed. They are more likely to backfire.

Although the physicians, therapists and other professionals who work with this clientele may be committed, caring people who make sincere efforts in their roles, they are so misled in their understanding of the problems they treat that, like their clients, their struggles usually bear little fruit.

Let's take a look at some specific eating problems, from the traditional descriptions as well as from some newer popular terms and definitions. This will help you identify your own symptoms and later, in Chapter 3, learn why you experience them.

EATING DISTURBANCES—WHAT'S WHAT?

Along with the traditional definitions of the best-known eating disorders, anorexia and bulimia, we'll discuss some popular descriptive labels: bulimarexia, compulsive undereating, compulsive overeating (including emotional overeating), food addiction and the new, broader term "eating disturbance."

Anorexia Nervosa

"Anorexia" simply means "without appetite," and "nervosa" means "mental in origin." This lack of appetite is the hallmark of anorexia, but it is a bit misleading. Although it appears that anorectics do not experience hunger because they eat so little, most do get hungry and at times their hunger is so extreme that it frightens them. Although anorectics experience mental symptoms, I believe these symptoms do not cause anorexia. Instead, they usually result from self-starvation.

Here's a checklist of the symptoms usually associated with anorexia. Check any symptom that applies to you.

Symptoms of Anorexia Nervosa
—Self-starvation, chronic undereating
—Obsession with being thin
—Refusal to maintain body weight within normal limits

—Weight loss 15 percent or more below normal limits
—Failure to gain weight appropriate for body growth
—Intense fear of gaining weight or becoming fat
—Body-image disturbance; a claim to feeling fat even though
  underweight or emaciated
—Absence of three consecutive menstrual cycles (without other
  cause)
—Abuse of laxatives and diuretics to control weight
—Purging of food by excessive exercise or self-induced vomit-
  ing after eating

*Marianne became concerned about her eating when she
was just twelve. About a year after she started to develop
breasts and hips, she saw a TV program about our country's
high-fat diet and abruptly decided to go low-fat in her own eating. At first she continued to eat with her family, avoiding fatty
foods, but after a while nothing her parents served was accept-
ably low-fat for her. She grew preoccupied with eating and
food preparation. She developed strict rules and standards for
food quality, gradually lowering the fat in her diet until it was
absent. She started jogging. Her appetite became erratic. She
skipped meals, sometimes going all day on a few rice cakes or
crackers. She lost weight. At five feet and 105 pounds, Marianne was never big to begin with, but she liked feeling smaller
because she felt more comfortable around her slim girlfriends.
This fueled her anti-eating and exercise efforts even more.*

*Marianne's parents began to argue with her, suggesting
that she eat a little more and relax her strict rules. Eventually
she wouldn't talk about her eating with anyone. She seemed
locked in a world of her own determination. Eight months
and twenty-two pounds later, Marianne seemed to have wan-
dered into a hopeless pattern, beyond help. She insisted she
was much too fat, but her bones were visible everywhere.*

Anorectics, like many other people with eating disturbances,
are usually "experts" on nutrition, capable of listing the calorie
and fat contents of dozens and sometimes hundreds of foods.
They talk, think, read and worry about food; and hoard it. Their
world revolves around the topics of food and eating while they
carefully and persistently avoid taking any substantial nourishment

into their bodies. They may even prepare elaborate meals for others, spending hours at the grocery store and in the kitchen, but then refuse even to taste their culinary creations. It is the intensity of their fear of weight gain, coupled with their success at avoiding food, that sets anorectics apart from those suffering from other eating struggles.

Bulimia

"Bulimia" means "a constant and insatiable craving for food." This extreme sensation of hunger causes anxiety and even panic for those who are fearful of becoming overweight because they know that satisfaction of this morbid hunger will lead to weight gain. Loss of control over their appetites triggers bulimic bingeing, and panic about gaining weight prompts purging. Many popular medical reference books refer to bulimia as an emotional disorder, but I haven't found that theory valid in my work.

Here's the symptoms checklist for bulimia or compulsive overeating. Check each symptom that applies to you.

Symptoms of Bulimia
—Strict dieting or fasting to control weight
—Recurrent episodes of binge eating (consuming large amounts of food in a short time)
—A loss of control over eating behavior
—Self-induced vomiting, use of laxatives or diuretics, vigorous exercise and/or use of amphetamines to control weight
—Preoccupation with diet, weight and body image
—Distorted body image

Like anorexia, the number-one symptom of bulimia is undereating—eating significantly less food than you need. Bulimics are just as afraid of being fat as anorectics, but they are less successful at staying away from food. They are determined to control their eating by strict food avoidance and often develop elaborate rules and systems, just like anorectics, but they lose control of their eating in spite of their determination and because of their misguided efforts. Compulsive overeaters have all the symptoms of bulimia, except they may not purge.

Bulimics may be underweight, overweight or of normal weight. Many bulimics have been anorectic, and vice versa.

Bulimarexia

This self-descriptive term is relatively new. One definition for "bulimarexia" is "a psychological disorder in which a person alternates between an abnormal craving for food and an aversion to it, found especially among young women." In my experience, this condition is always accompanied by strict dieting, food phobia and avoidance, and obsession with food and eating. It's really no more "psychological" than dieting! This term is often used interchangeably with anorexia or bulimia. More on bulimarexia at the end of this chapter.

THE COMMON DENOMINATOR IN EATING DISORDERS—DIETING

I have never met an overeater who wasn't also an undereater—eating *less* food than she needs at times. I have never met an undereater who wasn't afraid of food because of traditional diet propaganda: that eating less and food avoidance are the keys to weight control. Every eating disturbance that I have encountered in more than five hundred clients started with dieting. And I have observed that most typical dieters suffer from at least some symptoms of bulimia.

Linda began her dieting efforts rather innocently after her first baby was born. Just two weeks postpartum, she was still about thirty pounds overweight and fearful of never losing it, like her mother. So Linda joined Weight Watchers and enjoyed her early success—a ten-pound loss in just three weeks. This is easier than I thought it would be, she reflected. But two weeks later Linda found herself raiding the refrigerator in the middle of the night—Swiss cheese and mayonnaise and chips and ice cream. This raid happened nearly every night, although Linda had never been a nocturnal eater before. In spite of these binges, she lost twelve pounds. When she plateaued, she cut down even more on her meal portions. She tried skipping her snacks, drinking diet pop instead. But her weight wouldn't budge. "You must be cheating," her counselor accused her. She was cheating. She was eating less than she was supposed to be.

One meeting day about three months into her very hungry diet, Linda "weighed in" and the scale showed a two-pound gain. That did it. After the meeting she went straight to the bakery across the street and bought a dozen huge caramel sweet rolls that were full of pecans. Linda sat in her car and began to eat the pastries, one after another, in rapid succession. She ate every last one and felt like a giant caramel roll herself. She caught a glimpse of herself in the mirror with her cheeks stuffed to capacity and the caramel dripping down her chin. This is one of those binges, she thought. I'm becoming an emotional overeater. I got so upset about the weight gain that I stuffed myself.

Embarrassed to return to Weight Watchers, Linda decided to try cutting down on her own. She found staying away from food altogether even easier in some ways than controlled eating. So most of the day she just skipped any serious food and sipped low- or no-calorie drinks. The only problem was in the evening. Her hunger seemed to get the best of her then, and she often lost control of her appetite, overeating the worst foods possible: chips, dips, ice cream, cookies and peanut butter. Now and then Linda would eat an entire pan of brownies or fudge, driven by a compulsive urge that she didn't understand. As her weight increased gradually, Linda's efforts doubled and she began a round of local diet programs. It didn't matter what program she tried, sooner or later the bingeing would creep back in. She simply could not control it indefinitely. Finally, out of desperation, Linda joined Overeaters Anonymous, where she learned that she was "addicted to food."

With researchers and "experts" leading the way, we have developed some superficially logical psychological theories to explain bizarre eating patterns. Although anorexia and bulimia seem to be very mysterious and complicated (as psycho-emotional problems can be), and have historically been classified as mental disorders, I will explore a simpler formula behind the development of these disorders: a desire to be thin that leads to undereating that leads to eating disturbances. It is this simple equation that links all these sick eating patterns together and promises to shed new light on their common physical cause.

LOVE HUNGER OR FOOD HUNGER?

The symptoms of eating disturbances we've looked at never seem to develop in people who aren't trying to get or stay thin by ignoring their hunger and eating less food than they need. The desire to be thin that motivates undereating occurs in a culture which equates thinness with success and unilaterally rejects people who are overweight, so it's not too hard to understand why people want to be thin or fear weight gain. What may be hard for some people to understand is the degree of self-destruction to which a person will go on this road to a fat-free body.

Eating problems *appear* to be psycho-emotional in nature because, as many of us know, people with eating disorders can get so weird! But the eating disturbed really aren't as weird as they act, considering their dilemma. The physical nature of that dilemma is explored in Chapter 2.

It is the understandable desire for thinness, coupled with a gross misunderstanding about the real cause of weight gain, that sets highly motivated individuals up for bizarre eating patterns that threaten their health and vitality. Emotional troubles and unmet psychological needs are *not* at the heart of crazy eating habits. *Fear of food and undereating are.* People with eating problems may or may not have enough love in their lives, but one thing is certain: they do not have enough good food when they need it.

Compulsive Undereating

Although this term sounds suspiciously like a synonym for anorexia, it isn't. Compulsive undereating refers to the chronic urge to avoid food, eat less than you want or restrict your eating in other ways, in order to control weight. I have found that the label "compulsive undereater" usually applies to anyone who seriously adopts traditional diet principles, and this includes a huge population, especially women. Diet methods train individuals in compulsive undereating. And it is compulsive undereating that propels the vicious Feast or Famine Cycle (see Chapter 3), and all the eating disturbances associated with that cycle.

Compulsive Overeating and Emotional Overeating

These labels are used as a self-diagnosis by many who regularly lose control of their eating and overeat or binge compulsively, often in response to emotional stress. Overeaters Anonymous has helped make the term "compulsive overeater" popular, since members often use it to refer to their alleged addiction. The term is used interchangeably with "food addiction" (which is discussed in the next section, along with more about OA).

I have discovered a very interesting irony in counseling clients from this group. Compulsive overeaters are always very much aware of their overeating behavior and readily admit that it is a problem. Often the evidence is rather obvious. But these bingers just as certainly have another symptom which they almost never identify: compulsive undereating.

Compulsive overeaters rarely recognize that undereating is part of their disorder, but it is just as pathological as its opposite and actually lies at the root of the disturbed eating pattern. Because undereating, unlike overeating, doesn't show up on the body, it is harder to see as part of the problem. Besides, who would ever imagine that an overweight person could actually be eating *less* than she should? It doesn't seem to make sense until you really sit down and think it through, which is exactly what we're going to do in the next two chapters. The critical relationship between these two polar symptoms is the key to understanding eating disturbances.

But why do compulsive overeaters so often start a binge under the influence of heavy emotions? Isn't that proof that their eating disorder is psychological?

All people experience stressful emotions at times, but most don't overeat as a response because the natural physiological reaction to stress is a *loss* of appetite, not its stimulation. Eating is actually stressful to the body, and digestion will be delayed when more pressures are present. But this normal response is contingent on the eating habits of the individual, so that only when a person is well fed does the appetite tend to shut down under stress.

By contrast, when a person who is underfed suffers emotional stress, a paradox occurs. Rather than representing an additional stress to the body, eating for the underfed is a stress relief, promising to solve at least the chronic, underlying problem of inadequate fuel intake. So emotional problems and other forms of stress provoke chronic undereaters to eat and often overeat. Their bodies are simply using the stress as an opportunity for catching up on their inadequate eating.

Food Addiction

Many people consider themselves food addicted, usually as a result of their affiliation with Overeaters Anonymous. OA is an organization based on the same recovery principles as Alcoholics Anonymous. Instead of alcohol addiction, OA members deal with what they consider an addiction to food, which they also call compulsive overeating. The concept of food addiction is very appealing to many people whose eating behavior feels out of control, compulsive and impossible to explain. Many professionals are engaged in therapies based on this addiction model because they, too, see compulsive overeating and bingeing as inexplicable by another means.

The only problem with this approach is that it is completely unfounded and does nothing to help people normalize their eating behavior or their body weights. People find some much-needed camaraderie and support for their feelings of isolation and despair at OA meetings, but most of the ideas about eating control are superstitious and the counsel shared is typically unsubstantiated diet propaganda. I know I am desecrating a holy cow here because many dejected dieters are extremely loyal to OA. For them it has been the only place left to turn in the hopelessness of dietland failure. But along with positive stories of support, I have heard some alarming reports of OA tactics designed to motivate "food-addicted" members to stay away from food, based on theories that inspire even more fear in these already fear-ridden people.

If you really think you are, in a way somehow unlike normal people, addicted to a substance you must have every day in order to survive, you are doomed to a cycle of fear/control/avoidance/loss of control/fear. This cycle will be described and illustrated thoroughly in Chapter 3.

Everyone is addicted to food, and to air and water, for that matter. We would all suffer withdrawal symptoms if any of these substances was restricted below our needs. In fact, the withdrawal symptoms associated with food restriction are exactly what this book is about.

But why would some people think of themselves as food addicts in a special way? What makes this "diagnosis" seem so right? And what makes even professionals buy this food-addiction theory?

Eating Out of Control

People who consider themselves food addicted describe their symptoms: uncontrollable cravings for food (usually sweets and rich foods); bingeing or eating huge amounts of food at a time (usually forbidden food); obsession and preoccupation with food; fantasizing about food and eating; feeling "high" during or after food binges; depression and/or irritability during binges or periods of abstinence; terrible guilt about eating; inability to control eating once it gets started; inability to stay away from "bad" food; serious physical, emotional and social consequences of overeating. Doesn't this sound like "foodaholism"? Indeed it does, but it isn't. It just sounds like it.

There are physical reasons for these symptoms, which, by the way, are reported to some degree by most dieters. People who have these symptoms are no more food addicted than people who don't. The main difference between the two groups is this: people with these symptoms are trying to avoid eating a good part of the time and those without symptoms are eating. What's behind these so-called food-addiction symptoms will be discussed at length in Chapter 3.

Self-Check: What Have You Been Taught?

Check off any question that applies to you.

—Have you been told that your eating problems are about your dysfunctional family?

—Did anyone ever suggest that your mother's using food as a reward when you were a child caused your compulsive eating?

—Have you been "helped to discover" what purpose your extra fat plays in protecting you from something bad that happened in your past?

—Was it ever pointed out to you that your eating behavior is connected to your sexual hang-ups?

—Were you ever told that your overeating is about your fear of men? Of women? Of sex?

—Have you sought help for your disturbed eating patterns from a therapist and learned all sorts of interesting psychoemotional reasons for your disorder, such as every problem you ever had?

—Have you tried any spiritual remedies, such as prayer or meditation, for your eating problems?

—Have you been labeled a food addict, a foodaholic, a compulsive overeater, a glutton? Other words?

Has any of this helped you get your eating back to normal?
I didn't think so. It's been my experience that most people afflicted with eating struggles have psychological problems, and
sometimes serious ones. And virtually all, I have observed, suffer
emotional and mental consequences of their bizarre eating patterns. One universally cited symptom associated with eating disorders is anxiety—about food, about eating, about weight gain. That
certainly is a predominant psychological feature. But are rational
fears really symptoms? And is it abnormal for overly hungry people to have emotional distress over food?

OVEREATING—A SYMPTOM, NOT THE CAUSE

Overeating has been identified as the singular cause of weight
gain, and if it really is we are left to explain the cause of the overeating. Here is where all our colorful theories come in. What makes
people eat too much, especially when they know that overeating
will make them fat? Since everybody rejects fat people, it must be
something very powerful that compels a behavior that causes
weight gain. Aha! It must be deep-seated needs, like love. Or perhaps deep-seated hurts, like childhood trauma. Or maybe deep-
seated issues, like sexuality. Yes, these things could do it! And voilà!
The clients we counsel, one after another, just happen to have at
least one of these deep-seated problems. Aren't we smart?

I have discovered that overeating, by itself, is not the cause of
overweight but merely a symptom of an underlying problem. In
fact, overeating is a healthy, normal response to this problem: undereating. I believe that undereating provokes compensatory
overeating, preoccupation with food and all the symptoms of eating disturbance. These symptoms are really manifestations of
adaptation—the body's survival system—designed to keep body
and soul together under stressful environmental conditions. Lack
of food is one such condition that forces the body to make
changes, sometimes rather drastic ones, for survival's sake.

Undereating, food avoidance, portion control and meal-skip-
ping because of busy schedules all inspire the adaptive make-up
eating and preoccupation with food that we have all experienced.

There's nothing psychological about it until we start feeling guilty and ashamed about overeating. And that comes from a lack of understanding. If we only knew that food isn't really the problem but the solution we just might have a chance to get over our fear of eating and get on with developing a normal relationship with food. Wouldn't that be something? It's all coming up, so keep reading.

Almost every psychologist and psychiatrist whom I know of reflects a confidence in the theory that aberrant eating behavior is psychogenic in origin. In fact, every individual I have ever interviewed who had a history of an eating disorder has confirmed that she learned from professionals or from books that her trouble with eating was originally caused by, and continued because of, psychological disturbance. Not one, however, reported significant or lasting relief from symptoms as a result of psychological or behavioral therapies *as long as her undereating efforts continued.*

> *In her third year of college, Patti finally sought help for her long-standing struggle with bulimia. She was beginning to feel some serious physical effects—muscle weakness, heart palpitations, occasional light-headedness and trouble concentrating. The psychologist to whom Patti went, after two sessions that covered her family history, sexual development and relationships with men, told her that she was in a depression and suggested she see a psychiatrist for an anti-depressant medication.*
>
> *The next six months Patti went faithfully to her therapist. She took the anti-depressant and thought it made her feel better. She talked and talked about her feelings, dreams, hurts and struggles week after week. She never missed. Finally, the therapist began to gently explore with Patti the "significance" of her binge/purge behavior. She told Patti that repressed anger was often a trigger for bulimic behavior, and perhaps Patti would be interested in doing some "anger work." Then again, Patti had some sexual issues that might be coming out in her bulimia. Would she like to explore that possibility?*
>
> *Gradually, Patti felt better, at least emotionally. The medication was probably helping. Physically, she was dragging a bit and still eating and purging as crazily as ever. Little the counselor had said about her emotional problems really rang true to Patti, except maybe the anger with her father. But she just wasn't into it, so she quit.*

If eating problems really do have a psychological basis, why do almost all victims fail to gain lasting relief from their eating disturbances even after years of therapy? And how could so many individuals benefit so dramatically from a program, outlined in my first book, that is not psychological at all, but physical both in theory and in practical application? I am not implying that psychotherapy is not indicated or ever beneficial for some people when they suffer from disturbed eating, especially for other problem areas of life. It may be extremely helpful in some ways, but eating problems continue in spite of this progress when overall eating patterns are not addressed. I am suggesting that the theoretical connection between eating disorders and emotional problems is highly exaggerated, to the detriment of millions who suffer with eating afflictions.

EATING DISTURBANCES REDEFINED

The definition of eating disturbance that I use is this:

Any pattern of eating that interferes with a person's emotional, physical or social balance or health.

In other words, if your eating behavior or relationship with food is a problem for you, you have an eating disturbance. Of course, this definition would include the classic categories and the popular labels. Now forget all the technicalities that we've discussed before. Does this definition fit you? It's important to admit because that's the first step in getting well.

What's the Difference?

I have lumped all eating troubles together in my definition because I believe these disturbances all come from the same basic problem. All eating-disturbed people have several major symptoms in common and the most obvious one is abnormal eating behavior. The other symptoms they share, though not so apparent on the surface, are so similar that they ultimately blur the distinctions among the different categories. The evidence that best points to this breaking down of the distinctions between the classic eating disorders is the new term "bulimarexia."

If the main symptom of anorexia is lack of appetite, and the main symptom of bulimia is excessive appetite, then how can these disorders, which claim opposite central characteristics, possibly overlap? Isn't it remarkable that most anorectics also have symptoms associated with bulimia? Yes, it is. And is it just a coincidence that most bulimics also share the classic symptoms of anorexia? No, it isn't.

Flip Sides of the Same Coin

The term "bulimarexia" has been coined because anorexia and bulimia are flip sides of the same disorder. They share the same basic cause, which is undereating, and only a few symptoms separate these categories: degree of appetite experienced, success in controlling eating, and purging. But, as we've discovered, even these symptoms overlap. What's left to make these disorders separate? Not much.

The Connecting Cycle

Anorexia, bulimia, and all of the other eating disturbances described in this chapter are simply variations on the same cycle—the Feast or Famine Cycle. The interesting discoveries that come from this cycle model are (1) the similarity of the eating and behavior patterns among the different disturbances, (2) the obvious consistency of symptoms between eating disturbances and the cycle, and (3) the common origin—undereating—among all eating disturbances.

The Feast or Famine Cycle is propelled by conscious attempts to undereat for weight control or by unconscious undereating habits (i.e., when schedules interfere with the availability of food). You're about to discover the powerful effect this cycle has on your body, your eating and your emotional life. Armed with this information, you can finally learn to eat normally and start enjoying a long and happy relationship with food.

Prerequisites to Breaking Out

If you really want to get your eating problems solved, you've got to shake off the victim role of the dieter and accept the personal power you have to change what you can now. You can't change your history, but you can carve out a different future for yourself. This is not going to be easy. Change for human beings is never easy. But if you want your life to be free of eating disturbances, *you* have to eat differently—and you *can*.

CHAPTER 2

Understanding
Disturbed Eating:
The Famine Factor

Lauren was fifteen years old when dieting became her obsession and her eating avoidance crossed the line to anorexia. Hospitalized briefly at that time, she went back to eating more normally and began to gain weight. But when her clothes began to get tight Lauren panicked. She continued to eat more food in front of her family, but she learned to get rid of most of it by forcing herself to vomit.

Just before she turned eighteen, Lauren got a chance to model professionally. She tried to control her weight by strict dieting, but she began to binge more often. Purging became a necessary part of her life. At five feet ten and 110 pounds, Lauren was a fashion designer's dream, but she was living in a nightmare of the binge/purge cycle, laxative abuse, compulsive workouts, and constant anxiety about eating and weight gain. She usually ignored her symptoms—palpitations, muscle weakness, chronic fatigue, fainting spells, and dry skin and hair. Only the dry skin and hair really bothered her because she feared it might affect her career.

What is it about ultra-thinness that drives already thin young girls like Lauren to abuse their bodies like this, ignoring such serious danger signals?

Liz suffered through painstaking portion control and legalistic eating guidelines for over thirty years, off and on. This last round of dieting was nine months long, complete with a food scale and a human scale—both used many times daily. But the moment of victory was brief. Right after weighing in the day she reached her goal weight with Weight Watchers (in her thirty-second year of dieting, her sixth attempt with this organization), Liz found herself in front of the kitchen sink, cramming M&Ms down her throat faster than she could swallow them. As she looked at her reflection in the window, she told herself, "You have an eating disorder." The M&Ms were the beginning of the end of Liz's goal weight; it lasted exactly a day.

PATTERNS OF MISERY

Bulimics and compulsive overeaters often say their binges are overwhelming, sickening, confusing and frightening. Others report that they feel numb during binges, their emotions temporarily suspended. Nearly all say they feel out of control. Panic and powerful feelings of remorse always follow these food orgies, which may trigger purging in bulimics. The self-induced vomiting after a binge is often accompanied by more remorse, shame, guilt, anxiety—and some relief, they say, from the fear of weight gain. Purging by exercise looks healthier, but it's not. Like binge eating, exercise can become compulsive and extreme. Coupled with undereating and the binge/purge cycle, it is also physically debilitating.

Some anorectics' lives become so intolerable that they commit suicide before their self-starvation kills them directly. Some suffer permanent kidney or heart damage, and if they survive, usually continue to undereat. Anorectics and bulimics I have worked with share frightening tales of fainting and profound weakness from laxative and diuretic abuse. (Using chemical methods to get rid of the food they eat and the fluids they drink is common among anorectics and bulimics.) But their drug abuse doesn't usually stop even with these alarming signs of physical distress. People with eating disorders seem to be driven by demons.

Why would anyone like Lauren or Liz try to live on so little food that her eating patterns become bizarre and her health is endangered? And what's the difference between an anorectic like Lauren, who at the early stages is able to stay in control of her eating for months, and the bulimic or "food addict" like Liz, who can only manage undereating for limited periods before losing control? Why do some anorectics actually starve themselves to death?

Why don't more people starve themselves to death? Why is bulimia or compulsive overeating so much more common than anorexia? And why do eating-disordered people put up with such a tremendous amount of pain, frustration and physical problems, and still continue their crazy eating patterns? Can they help it? Are they really out of control? It surely looks as if they're mentally ill. Are they? These are all questions we'll be looking at in the coming chapters.

What About You?

Most people in food jail wonder about their own mental health.

Here are some questions to help you take a look at your own eating patterns and relationship with food. Don't panic over your answers. We have to take a look at food jail before we can break out of it!

—I'm afraid to eat, afraid of my own hunger.
—My appetite feels so huge that it makes me avoid food.
—Sometimes I eat in a compulsive, overwhelmed way.
—When I skip meals I always overeat later in the day.
—I often have strong cravings for chocolate, ice cream, fried foods or other rich treats.
—I can go without much food for so long, and then I overeat.
—I have to get really psyched up to be around party food.
—My eating seems to be automatic at times, as though I am driven to eat without my conscious consent.
—Since I was young I have never been able to maintain any weight loss.
—If I gain even a pound I panic.
—I find myself thinking about food much of the day.
—My friends say I'm thin, but I *feel* so fat.
—I'm afraid if I start eating I won't be able to stop.
—I have strict rules for myself about eating.
—I can only maintain my weight through rigidly controlled eating patterns.
—My appetite seems to be beyond satisfaction. Even when I eat, I never feel really satisfied.
—I wonder how other people can eat without even giving it a thought.
—If I stopped controlling my eating, I'd probably gain a hundred pounds.

—If there were a "thin pill" that was guaranteed to keep me svelte no matter what I ate but definitely increased the risk of cancer, I would take it.

—If I didn't binge, I wouldn't have to purge by making myself vomit, but I always end up bingeing.

—I don't know how normal people eat within their appetites. It's just beyond me.

How did you do? If you checked three or more, you absolutely must keep reading. But if you didn't find yourself in this list at all, there must be a friend whom you recognize, so keep reading anyway.

YOUR DISTURBED EATING STARTED WITH DIETING

I went through two periods of anorexia during my dieting years. These were punctuation periods in the more chronic condition I had—bulimia. Bulimic symptoms developed as my dieting took hold as a young teenager. I wasn't even overweight when I started dieting; I just thought I was. As I tried to control my eating I began to lose control of it, and started to overeat and binge, especially at night. So I tried to restrict my eating even more, and the binges grew more frequent and more extreme. I lost weight, I gained it back. My eating felt out of control much of the time. I developed a fear of food and started hating my body. I began to exercise in order to burn off calories and change my shape. I pored over diet books and articles for better control tactics. My life revolved around my weight and my diet. By the time I was fifteen I had become so thin and obsessive about my weight that I was hospitalized for tests.

My eating disorder developed from dieting. I've discovered that, with rare exception, eating disturbances always do. In eight years of counseling in this field I have never heard a significant variation on this basic story. For some people it's a different trigger behind the first diet efforts—a minor weight problem, a comment from a family member or friend, or a good experience with a body change from exercise. It doesn't matter. The eating disturbance may become more extreme or less. It doesn't matter. There may be a serious weight problem or an underweight problem, or any body size in between. It doesn't matter. Whatever gets a person started on dieting in the first place and how far into eating problems it takes her, it's dieting that inspires all the troubles that follow, whether great or small.

Dieting (or undereating) is the setup for eating disturbances.

After fifteen years of dieting with bulimic eating patterns, I became deeply discouraged. I realized that I had more than a weight problem, I had a lifestyle problem. My life was not my own. I had become almost completely obsessed with my weight, my eating, my body shape, how my clothes fit, exercising and, of course, dieting. I was miserable—overweight, underweight and all points in between. My weight was never stable since I was always losing pounds or gaining them back. My appetite was chronically huge and threatening, regardless of my body shape, and had to be constantly under the guard of my willpower, and fear.

Looking for clues to my weight and eating problems, I decided to study weight control. When I began to search for some understanding of the self-made hell I was in, I considered my appetite my arch enemy. I had no idea that my dieting efforts had anything to do with my disturbed eating behavior. I felt defective—unique in a bad way, and alone. I didn't talk about my bizarre eating with anyone. I was too ashamed. I did talk to hundreds of people of all shapes and sizes about their eating, and their dieting, experiences. And I discovered some extremely interesting new things.

UNDEREATERS ANONYMOUS

The most important discovery I made was this: Overweight people are *not* overeating all the time—they're *undereating* much of the time! In fact, all the overweight people I interviewed, dieters and nondieters alike, were trying to eat *less* a lot of the time in an effort to control their weight. And all people with disturbed eating—overweight, normal weight and underweight—were doing the same thing because they were trying to lose weight or they were afraid of gaining. Just like the obesity researchers, they all believed that eating too much is the cause of overweight, so they were all trying to eat less food.

Here it is, the revelation of the decade: *Overweight people are eating-avoidant.* And normal or underweight people who are afraid of becoming overweight are also eating-avoidant. I knew it was true, too, because I was afraid to eat whether I was fat or thin, and consequently I was avoiding food most of the time myself. The whole diet lifestyle is based on trying to eat less than you want. I began to question the very foundation of my life—dieting.

Another theme I heard over and over again from most typical waist watchers was this: At some point in their efforts to eat less, most undereaters reported losing control of the amount and type of food they ate. They usually blamed themselves and their emotions for this loss of control, but it was so common that I knew something was behind it besides lack of willpower. I didn't dismiss these reports of loss of control as excuses, as many researchers do, because these things were happening to me, too. I was trying to eat less chronically, and I was also losing control of my portions and food choices at times. But why?

Questions began to pop into my mind in the middle of the night: If people are trying *not* to eat so much of the time, why do so many overeat and gain weight over time? And how does all this undereating affect the body? The appetite? How do eating disturbances fit into this whole scheme? Is there something that ties these patterns together? Are we missing something here?

THE MISSING LINK

This is the revelation that kept surfacing and that eventually revolutionized my ideas about eating problems:

There is a potent biological correlation between under-eating and overeating.

With rare exception, people who undereat always, sooner or later, overeat, too. People who starve always eventually binge. Most dieters and undereaters can stay in control of their food avoidance for only limited periods, and when they lose control and start eating again, they always gain back lost weight—that is, unless they resort to purging, which seems to be the only way to beat the statistics. Restricted eating is followed by excessive eating, eating avoidance is followed by make-up eating, famines are always followed by feasts. The only people for whom these princi-

ples do not always apply are terminally ill, born with zero famine
sensitivity (a rare condition defined later in this chapter) or
anorectic. And many anorectics follow these patterns, too.

When undereaters lose control of their eating behavior, what is
in control? What has the power to take over the controls for something as basic as eating? Only one thing—the survival instinct.

AIR, WATER, FOOD

Three things in the physical environment are essential for staying alive: air, water and food. When our bodies are threatened
with their lack, our survival instincts and the adaptations they inspire step in to protect us from harm.

Mary, a normally benevolent and mild-mannered woman, was
reported to have broken the nose of an intruder who tried to suf-
focate her. Mary's behavior under these circumstances would not
be considered psychologically inspired, it would be viewed as
simple self-defense, motivated by the survival instinct.

Water Conservation

People who are stranded without water retain the fluid in their
bodies to prevent dehydration. This physical adaptation happens
quite automatically under the influence of hormones. Once the
level of fluid intake falls off, the body responds by recycling its
fluid reserves, wasting only the minimal amount of water in urine
and perspiration.

When people don't drink enough fluids to stay properly hy-
drated for any reason, they tend to retain water in their tissues.
The same protective mechanism is at work. When these underhy-
drated but bloated individuals complain to their doctors about
their puffiness, guess what the professionals recommend? "Drink
more water."

More water? That's right. People who are retaining fluid because
they don't drink enough need to drink more so their bodies can
stop protecting them from dehydration by holding on to fluid in
their muscles and soft tissue. And when they start drinking enough,
their bodies let go of the excess fluid that's been in storage.

What has all this got to do with eating problems? We've established the fact that people with eating problems are all trying to
eat less than their bodies are demanding. Their food supply is

threatened. When these undereaters develop huge appetites and cravings, and sometimes lose control of their eating and start to overeat and binge on all the "wrong" foods, they are confused and bewildered, but the explanation is quite simple: their survival instincts have taken over.

UNDEREATING—THE SURVIVAL TRIGGER

When people are determined to lose weight by eating less than their bodies need, a great power stands between them and their goal—their bodies' survival instinct. And when people try to keep from gaining weight by undereating (ignoring hunger, controlling portions, etc.), this survival mechanism is triggered and their bodies usurp eating controls, intensifying the appetite, producing cravings, conserving calories and forcing fat-producing food intake to prevent starvation.

Our bodies are equipped with powers even beyond our conscious willpower to override decisions we make that conflict with our survival. Traditional calorie-restricted diets and even our informal undereating habits threaten our survival and therefore backfire. If they didn't fail, many more of us would diet ourselves to death. But here we are, alive, undereating and overeating on a roller coaster.

I am not implying that diets don't "work," at least in a very limited way. They do cause weight loss, but for almost everyone, only temporarily. That's why many people, even those who have lost twenty pounds twenty different times, keep dieting to maintain or produce weight loss! They have lost weight on diets in the past, and they don't know what else to do.

And most undereaters (except some anorectics) eventually lose control of their eating, no matter how motivated they are, how much they want to be thin, how much medical supervision they have, how much behavior modification training they receive, how rich or famous they are. Losing control for undereaters isn't about willpower or education, money or fame, emotions or family issues—it's about staying alive.

After gaining fifteen pounds during her freshman year at college, Margaret returned home for the summer, worked full-time at a bank, and joined Weight Loss Clinic, determined to get back into shape. Her main goals were to save money, lose weight and play plenty of tennis during her three-month break.

During her lunch hour Margaret went to her Weight Loss Clinic, where she was given the basic diet plan on her second visit and paid for her first month. The fee included "medical supervision." A very thin young woman in a white coat took her blood pressure and weighed her. Margaret had never been on a formal diet before and she listened carefully as her "counselor" told her about the diet. She received an 800 calorie-a-day allowance that told her what to eat, exactly how much and when. It didn't sound like much food to Margaret, but she knew it was healthy—fruit, salads and lean meat and fish. She liked the friendly counselor, who told her that she had unlimited visiting privileges at the clinic. She could come in to be weighed or to talk anytime. She would get her money's worth, she vowed.

The first few days Margaret was quite hungry, so she drank a lot of water and other "unlimited drinks" from her diet card to help ease the emptiness. The fifth day she felt a little faint at work at around eleven in the morning and cheated on her diet for the first time. She had a milk shake from McDonald's. She had never had one before in her life, but she just felt she had to have it. When Margaret weighed in the next day, she was nervous. Four pounds! I've lost four pounds already! Hey, this isn't so bad. I even cheated!

The next few weeks were a tug-of-war. Margaret fought to stay fairly close to the diet limits, but her appetite seemed to be getting the best of her more and more often. She was definitely developing a sweet tooth, and really overeating now and then. Even at school she'd never had these strong cravings. Margaret was getting discouraged, especially after her one-month visit. She had lost only six pounds total. She knew why it wasn't more—she wasn't sticking to the diet—so she decided to get serious.

And she did. Margaret forced herself to stick rigidly with the 800 calories a day and also played tennis nearly every day. Her counselor had suggested that more aerobic exercise might help her lose faster and settle her appetite down. She was right. After the second month Margaret had lost sixteen pounds—ten pounds the second month alone. She was elated, *and even though she had already reached her goal weight, she decided to lose a few more pounds for insurance.*

Just a week later, though, Margaret fell on the tennis court and sprained her ankle badly. The doctor said she'd have to stay off it completely for a few weeks. She could use crutches to get around the house, but she had to keep the foot elevated most of the time. "Well, there go my tennis workouts," she complained. Although Margaret was disappointed, she was secretly glad for a chance to rest before going back to school. She was exhausted.

During the two weeks that Margaret was laid up she gained six pounds. Of course she wasn't doing much physically, but her eating just seemed to be uncontrollable. She couldn't get her mind off food. Every day for a week she promised herself she'd stick to her diet, and every day she found herself overeating by afternoon. Her appetite seemed unquenchable. By the second week, she gave up: the conflict ended as she gave in to her appetite. Margaret rested her ankle and ate until she went back to college.

By the time she got to school Margaret had gained back ten of the sixteen pounds she'd lost. She thought of the $300 she had spent on her diet—money she needed for school. By Christmas break, she had gained ten more pounds, in spite of her continuing efforts to diet and exercise. That fall Margaret learned from a friend how to "recover" from a binge by vomiting, but even that didn't keep her from gaining. All told, Margaret gained twenty pounds following the sixteen she had lost. For all her time, effort, money, pain and struggle, she netted a four-pound gain, plus an eating disorder.

Margaret's story is not unique. Hundreds of dieters have shared their undereating histories with me. And, like Margaret, they all felt hopeless and trapped. If you're like them, take heart. Your body is not defective. In fact, you're about to find out how very "successful" it really is.

SURVIVAL AND ADAPTATION

The scientific concept of adaptation describes how different species adjust to changes in the environment in order to survive.

Human beings, as well as animals, are equipped with many elaborate systems that support survival in the widely varied and ever-changing environments on earth. There are many common examples of adaptation, including the pigmentation of the skin with sunlight exposure (tanning effect) and the fluid retention that accompanies water restriction described earlier. Adaptive responses are built into organisms to preserve health and life, but sometimes they are misunderstood. Excess fat accumulation on human bodies is an example of adaptation that has been completely misunderstood.

FAT: FOOD STORED FOR SURVIVAL

Fat on human bodies was not always considered the villain it is today in developed countries. Historically, heavier people, especially buxom women, were regarded as healthier, wealthier and even wiser. Underweight (or what we now consider normal), particularly for women at different periods in history, was thought undesirable and a liability for attracting a husband. How times have changed!

Times may have changed, but our bodies' survival instincts haven't. The fact is, fat has always been an extremely important survival aid. It is not the curse of nature we have learned it is, so get ready to think of fat in a brand-new way. This new perspective will shed some much-needed light on the mystery behind your eating problems.

EXTRA BODY FAT—WHO NEEDS IT?

Before modern methods of food preservation and storage, people experienced natural variations in the availability of food, usually in yearly cycles. Sometimes periods of famine or plenty spanned even longer periods. In order to have enough fuel to survive when the outside food supply fell below maintenance levels, the human body had to have the capacity to store fuel inside itself—and it did. Human bodies stored fat for the future during times of abundance, and this stored fuel was used later during lean times. Famine-imposed undereating was counterbalanced by overeating and fat storage during times of plenty. In fact, it was the famine experience itself that provoked excessive eating and adaptive fat storage during higher food availability, in preparation for future famines.

Well, we don't have real famines now, at least not in our country, so we don't need these archaic food storage systems anymore, right? Wrong.

Most famines in our country today come in the form of willful undereating. All kinds of people are undereating for different reasons, and by these undereating efforts, they're inadvertently training their bodies to need to store more fat for future famines! This is why, with all our dieting and food avoidance, we're getting fatter and fatter as a nation. Eating disorders are epidemic for the same reason.

So basically, extra body fat and the mechanisms that promote fat storage keep people alive when they don't, for various reasons, eat enough. This implies that overweight people aren't eating enough when they should! The ability to store and maintain extra body fat is an adaptive trait because it's there to protect bodies from starvation. Based on these observations about the important role that fat plays in survival, I redefined excess weight gain:

Excess fat accumulation is an adaptive response to an environment where food is intermittently restricted.

When we limit our eating below our bodies' needs, we create the environment that promotes fat storage and sets up a war with our own survival instincts! Consequently, getting thinner or staying that way cannot be accomplished by working against our bodies' instincts, without developing eating problems. And eating disturbances cannot be effectively treated without dealing with undereating behavior and the attitudes and beliefs that compel it.

Undereating "hooks" the body's survival instincts and provokes adaptive responses that lead to weight gain. People in this trap usually respond to these adaptive urges by tightening the controls on their eating and/or wasting the food they eat (through exercise, vomiting or drug abuse). In response to this even more severe famining, the body adapts further: the appetite surges, the metabolism slows even more, cravings for rich foods intensify, panic ensues.

The survival conflict created by willful undereating is the true basis of eating disturbances.

Is it possible to end this conflict? How can we stop triggering this survival response and get permanent control of our hunger?

Ah, there's that fearful word—hunger. Why can't we get control of it? And why has our hunger gone berserk—become extreme, erratic, compelling, absent, controlling, distorted? It's almost evil.

APPETITES OFF THE DEEP END

People with eating disturbances have bizarre appetites that don't seem to be designed to do anything positive. In fact, the one symptom that all eating-disturbed people have in common is an extreme appetite that takes its victim hostage. What's adaptive about that? What has gone so terribly wrong in the bodies of people with eating disturbances?

When food intake is restricted for any reason, most bodies adapt by conserving energy and eventually accumulating fat to prepare for the possibility of a future famine. Remember, these bodies develop a need for fat to survive times of famine. The underlying problem in eating disturbances is that the food supply of the undereater is uncertain since "famines" occur regularly. Eating-disturbed people all experience either chronic or intermittent food restriction because of their commitment to weight control. It has precious little to do with psychology and everything to do with biology.

THE BEAR FACTS

The Science Museum of Minnesota produced a wonderful exhibit on bears a few years ago that illustrates the biological influence on eating behavior. The following observations are taken from the exhibit on hibernation.

Grizzlies and black bears prepare for hibernation [or famine] with a bout of frenzied feeding or hyperphasia. They might feed for up to 20 hours and consume 20,000 calories a day—about five times their normal intake. [Can you relate to this?] They become very fat, but they have consumed, almost to the calorie, the amount of energy they need [to survive] during hibernation.

The fattest bears hibernate first, the thinner bears continue to eat as long as food is available.

Scientists have concluded that hibernation is a biochemically controlled phenomenon. This means that the overeating, fat storage and use of excess fat during winter hibernation are internally controlled and inspired.

So, bears binge. They are biologically programmed to seasonal gluttony. In my opinion, bears don't overeat because of emotional problems or stress. People don't either.

HOW DOES A BODY DO IT?

At least five specific adaptive mechanisms at work keep under-eaters alive. These adaptive responses, inspired by undereating, are responsible for the hunger havoc and other symptoms that eating-disturbed people experience. Here's a list of the main adaptive responses that promote fat storage when a body doesn't get enough food:

1. lowered metabolic rate
2. increased appetite and/or urge to overeat or binge, often with some loss of control over eating behavior
3. high interest in, and cravings for, fat-producing foods (especially sweets and fatty foods)
4. preoccupation with food and eating
5. depressed interest in physical activity

These are the basic responses of any body when confronted with either chronic or intermittent food restriction. People whose appetites are exaggerated are or have been eating less quality food than they need. Generally, as eating decreases below survival limits, the appetite increases to compensate. But this adaptation doesn't always occur immediately following a period of undereating. In fact, it is sometimes delayed by days, weeks or even months, especially when the determination to limit eating is very high.

By the way, a world hunger relief organization cited the minimum nutritional requirement of an average adult to be 2,100 calories a day to maintain weight and health. Every dieter I have ever coached considered this amount far too many calories to eat in a day, even for maintenance! And it's considered a *minimum* adult caloric requirement in developing countries. Guess what? It's a good guideline for us to figure just about where these survival responses are going to get triggered. For most adults, except the most sedentary or elderly, any diet under 2,100 calories a day signals potential starvation to the body. From my experience in this field, that includes every single diet I've ever encountered or heard about. Even so-called higher-calorie diets are inadequate, and therefore threatening to the body.

With this guideline for "starvation" in mind, let's look at each of these five ways that bodies adapt to undereating.

1. Lowered Metabolic Rate:

Did you know that your metabolism (body combustion rate) drops when you eat less than you need? That's right. In fact, researchers have estimated that it drops significantly, between 15 and 30 percent! This means that dieting efforts, or eating avoidance, cause the body to conserve calories, to become more energy efficient, because the undereating is perceived by the body as a threat—a fuel-supply threat. Your body doesn't know you're trying to eat less. It doesn't care, either. All your body knows is what it gets, and if the food it gets isn't enough it turns its burners down. This metabolic rate adjustment makes much better sense when you consider what the body is trying to accomplish. It looks like pure sabotage but it isn't, because bodies just can't distinguish between a true famine and an artificial one.

2. Increased Appetite and/or Urge to Overeat or Binge, Often with Some Loss of Control over Eating Behavior:

The powerful urges to overeat and binge are adaptations to undereating. Overeating and bingeing are provoked by the exaggerated appetite commonly experienced by undereaters. The need for fat in underfed bodies translates directly to the appetite-control mechanisms that produce the urge to consume excessive amounts of food. This happens irrespective of the amount of fat already accumulated. Bodies don't have a "fat-o-stat," so even overweight people who undereat at times provoke their bodies' adaptive need for more fat with an intensified appetite. Significant overeating and the urge to overeat, I have observed, occur only in people who are, or have been, undereating.

Julie drank a glass of diluted juice on her way to work every day. She just wasn't that hungry; besides, she was watching her weight. Mineral water and tea helped hold her until lunchtime, if she could resist the donuts at the office. Then she usually had soup and a salad with low-cal dressing. But the major hunger really hit her in the afternoon—her "danger zone," as she called it. Sometimes she would buy a box of pastries "for the staff," and then eat half of them herself. Or when there was an office birthday party she typically finished a whole cake off—frosting first. If she got through the danger zone without losing control, she was OK until about ten at night. Some nights she couldn't stop eating until she was actually sick. Purging after her binges seemed like the only way to keep herself from gaining even more weight. She had no idea why she just couldn't control her appetite.

3. High Interest in, and Cravings for, Fat-Producing Foods (Especially Sweets and Fatty Foods):

Dieters don't crave broccoli. This isn't just a coincidence. Dieters and other undereaters tend to crave sweet and/or fatty foods. Researchers have even documented a correlation between dieting and increased cravings for high-calorie mixtures of sugar and fat because the body of an undereater is influenced by the physiological need to store fat. Broccoli just isn't that great a raw material for fat production, but ice cream sundaes, pastries and potato chips surely are. We've known for some time that cravings are somehow linked to our nutritional needs. This principle holds true when undereaters want all those "bad" foods, too. In light of their bodies' needs, these rich foods are perfect for them.

But *why* don't undereaters crave nutrient-rich foods, like vegetables, whole-grain cereals, skim milk and fruit? The answer is simple—priorities. The body's top survival priority in a famine environment is fat storage because, without enough food to stay alive, a body's nutritional status doesn't count for much. If you're dead from starvation, does it really matter how nutrient-rich your diet has been recently?

But don't undereaters need nutrients from quality foods, too?

Yes, they do, but most nutrient-rich foods tend to be lower in fat and refined sugar, and consequently don't qualify for the necessary fat-producing qualities that famine protection demands. So your cravings for fat producers mean you're not eating enough good food when you need it. It's a simple and infallible truth.

4. Preoccupation with Food and Eating:

Underfed people, whether overweight, underweight or of normal weight, think more about food than people who eat enough. Preoccupation is an adaptive response, not a psychological one, because, if we really are in danger of starving to death, and food comes along but we aren't paying attention, we might succumb before we'd think to eat something. All food-deprived humans, even naturally thin ones, become preoccupied with it.

Why am I so sure about this? When undereaters I've coached learn to eat enough good food whenever they get hungry, they invariably lose this preoccupation with food.

Larry, a friend of mine, read Fit for Life *and decided to try the program: fruit for breakfast, salad for lunch, properly combined protein and vegetables for supper. It sounded healthy and Larry wanted to increase his energy and stamina. The authors said he would. He tried to eat according to the recommendations for two years. Then he called me.*

Larry had been naturally thin for thirty years before he read Fit *and now he had an eating disorder. He was confused and worried. Since he started the Fit Diet (as I like to call it, since it causes fits of hunger), he had become obsessed with food and eating. He also struggled with intense hunger that led to bingeing and had developed cravings for fatty foods that he couldn't seem to resist. These were problems he'd never had before in his life.*

I pointed out the connection between his inadequate diet and his preoccupation and cravings. Then I explained what was happening to his body and that these symptoms were completely reversible. Larry was very relieved. He went back to his more relaxed eating patterns—a healthful variety of foods on demand—and within two weeks his "eating disorder" had disappeared.

5. Depressed Interest in Physical Activity:

Should a starving body be eager to waste calories in unnecessary physical activity? It isn't adaptive for bodies that are in danger of starving to demonstrate a hearty appetite for exercise. In fact, undereating and exercise are not compatible, at least not in survival terms. We certainly have tried to make these incongruent activities an integral part of our lifestyle, but it isn't working because it violates our bodies' number-one job—keeping us alive. Food-restricted dieting, by itself, is quite hard on the body, forcing multiple physiological adjustments, but the latest craze of dieting with regular workouts is even more blatantly suicidal. No wonder dieting exercisers have such high drop-out rates. Few bodies are designed to put up with such insanity, and few bodies actually do.

Bulimarectics are known for their "purging by exercise" behavior. People with eating problems sometimes believe they must work out to force their bodies to burn off food rather than store it. (There may be some truth to this for undereaters because of their adaptive need for fat storage.) This belief causes great anxiety about exercise—an emotional stress. Plus, the combination of undereating and overexercise is extremely stressful to the body—low-fuel supply plus high-fuel demand. To maintain such a strenuous regimen requires great determination and will, and what is the physical and personal cost of this lifestyle?

Undereaters usually don't *feel* like working out. This is adaptive. If the food supply is limited, the body needs to conserve energy, not waste it. This is why undereaters often suffer from chronic low energy and may not feel like "doing" anything physical. In fact, they commonly have a powerful urge to sit. At times, anorectics lack energy for even the modest physical activities of daily living because of their starvation state, but they, like bulimics, force themselves to exercise, even under the influence of this powerful biological reluctance. Although anorectics may experience a "high" at times, which they describe as stimulating, more often they have a chronic activity aversion that they must violate in order to work off those threatening calories through exercise. Their bodies are trying to get through to them, but they aren't listening. They're too scared.

DEFECTIVE BODIES OR DESTRUCTIVE DIETS?

Underfed bodies that need fat know how to accumulate it all by the five adaptive responses listed on pages 45. Since people with these symptoms don't understand what's happening, they usually interpret these adaptive responses as evidence that they have defective bodies. They don't understand why their appetites are so big, or why they crave rich, nutrient-poor foods, or why they always feel cold and unmotivated, or why they obsess about food all day long. Some people just figure they have a bad body—one that's determined to make them fat for no good reason. Others learn that there's something wrong with their psyches to explain their symptoms. Neither group has any idea of their bodies' real struggles or the part they themselves play in causing these symptoms.

These five symptoms are not built-in defects but the body's mechanisms for getting the fat it needs. Did you notice that these five adaptive responses perfectly parallel some classic symptoms of eating disorders? It's no coincidence.

Self-Check for Your Body's Adaptive Responses
Check any item you can relate to:

____ 1. My hands and feet are often cold.
____ 2. I feel chilled when others are comfortable.
____ 3. Although I eat less than others, I gain weight easily.
____ 4. The only way to maintain my weight is to carefully restrict my food intake.
____ 5. Once I let up even a little on my willpower, I usually overeat.
____ 6. I avoid situations where food is free and abundant.
____ 7. Nights are the worst for me—I lose control then.
____ 8. My body's "full" signal is out of order.
____ 9. I often overeat when I eat out.
____ 10. I buy sweets for others but eat them myself.
____ 11. My sweet tooth is famous.
____ 12. I have an intimate relationship with chocolate (or chips, or ice cream, etc.).
____ 13. I can eat low-fat foods just so long, and then I go berserk on fatty foods.
____ 14. At times it's hard to concentrate—to get food off my mind.

_____ 15. No one would ever know, but I think about food almost all day long.

_____ 16. I hate food—it haunts me.

_____ 17. Even going for a walk feels like too much at times.

_____ 18. My motivation seems to have deteriorated.

_____ 19. I hate sports/exercises that I once enjoyed.

_____ 20. Exercise is never fun anymore, it's work.

Dieters with moderate eating disturbances often gain weight under the influence of the five adaptive responses. As a matter of fact, the diet industry is established and maintained for the purpose of helping people overcome these responses—by teaching undereating techniques—but these symptoms are caused by undereating! So diet companies have more prospective customers now than ever before because they are promoting the problem they are promising to fix. Dieters lose weight and gain it back in a cycle pattern because of this irony, and many gradually gain back more weight than they are able to diet off. By the time they are in their late thirties or early forties, these double-decade diet veterans are not only battle weary, they are usually also heavier than ever. Just how these five adaptive responses fit into the cycle of weight loss and gain is discussed in Chapter 3.

If undereating is the environmental stress that provokes adaptive weight gain, the logical way to eliminate this need for extra fat, and the body's adaptive responses that produce it, is *to eliminate undereating.* This means that we have to learn to stop going hungry. We have to stop trying to limit our eating and *start learning to eat.* This is very difficult for people with eating fears. It is also the focal point for getting well, coming up in Chapters 4 to 6.

BODIES KNOW HOW TO BE THIN

Getting or staying thin must be done in harmony with our survival instincts if we want to be thin and enjoy normal eating habits, too. And it can be done! The most liberating discovery I made in researching obesity and eating disorders is this: You can eat plenty of good food whenever you get hungry and be thin, too. In fact, this is the only way to be "naturally thin," with normal eating patterns. I am convinced, from my own experience and twelve years of research and counseling hundreds of others, that the human body is designed to maintain a lean adapted body weight when it gets enough good food on demand.

Excess fat is always adaptive when a body is subjected to intermittent famines, or periods of undereating. Since extra fat is maladaptive for bodies that are consistently well fed, these bodies actually resist putting on weight! People who are naturally thin are prime examples. They have reputations for being the biggest and most frequent eaters, and their weight always stays about the same. As long as there is no survival need for extra fat, their bodies actually work to keep it to a healthy minimum.

What a concept! Our bodies will actually cooperate with us in staying thin if we will learn to eat enough of the right stuff.

THEY CAN DO IT, WHY CAN'T WE?

A small percentage of undereaters seem to be able to keep their weight down without eating problems. They just carefully limit their food intake and sometimes avoid "bad food" and stay thin. Moderate undereating seems to work for some people. Is that possible? Yes. Here's why.

HOW MUCH CAN A BODY TAKE: FAMINE SENSITIVITY

How readily your undereating efforts lead to eating disturbances depends on several critical factors. The most obvious one, of course, is the severity of your eating avoidance—how far your undereating goes. The range is broad, from anorectic fasting (which may not even include water) to moderate-calorie or fat-gram restriction. I call the level of food in the environment (which is considered edible to the individual) the "food availability factor," or FAF. Next, your activity level plays an important role. The higher the activity level in an undereater, the more severe the famine. Other factors that influence your body's peculiar response to undereating include your age, height and weight, stress level and hormones. The FAF, activity and stress levels are environmental, coming from outside the body. The internal aspects are about your unique physiology at your stage in life. But is anything in particular inherited about eating problems?

FOOD AVAILABILITY AND FAMINE SENSITIVITY

Obesity was once considered a function of environmental factors alone—too much food and too little exercise. But recently researchers are acknowledging that their simplistic stand on weight problems does not explain many cases and certainly hasn't led to any successful long-term solutions. So lately they have focused more on the inheritable traits that set certain people up for obesity and weight-control struggles.

We know that overweight is not inherited per se, but there is strong evidence that the predisposition to excess weight gain is definitely inherited from one's parents. I call this predisposition "famine sensitivity." It refers to those inherited traits that physically set a person up to gain weight easily under the influence of intermittent famines. Famine sensitivity plays an important role in the development of eating disturbances. That's why I'm going to ask you to do a simple self-assessment in the next section.

Some people have low famine sensitivity. In other words, their bodies are not especially tuned in to the food supply. They can eat recklessly, eat late, ignore their hunger at times, and their bodies do not respond by adjusting appetite levels and metabolic rates in order to add fat for survival insurance. They just stay lean, in spite of these periods of undereating. Usually they are young and from families where overweight is mild and rare. Sometimes, though, low-famine sensitives do not tolerate going hungry very well, so their famines, when they occur, are rather mild and short-lived.

Quite a few anorectics I have worked with, although certainly not all, have low famine sensitivity. Perhaps this is one factor that predisposes some people to developing anorexia—the natural physical ability to tolerate famining without losing control. Their bodies are naturally very lean and designed with a lower reaction quotient to undereating, tending to do fairly well with minimal food intake. Somehow, though, those who become anorectic feel they are never thin enough, and they learn to take advantage of their bodies' natural affinity for tolerating undersatisfied hunger. Anorectics with low famine sensitivity appear to be the most vulnerable to starving themselves to death because of these traits.

Fortunately, because it protects most undereaters from suicide, low famine sensitivity is not nearly as common as higher levels. Most people have higher famine sensitivity, and almost everybody's goes up as she gets older. We in the majority are more sensitive to going hungry—we have bodies that respond like lightning to undereating. Our fat-producing biochemicals seem to be lying in wait for their orders. We skip breakfast because we got up late, and vroom, the fat producers rev into gear to protect us and store up for the next day. We try that 1,000-calorie diet we read about in the rag mag and two days later we find ourselves overcome with bingeing at the bakery. We try adding thirty minutes of exercise to our new low-fat eating program and bang, we can't stop thinking about ice cream, or brownies, or betties or cobblers! Our bodies are out to protect us, and they're doing a mighty fine job.

People with higher famine sensitivity have to eat better than those with lower FS in order to escape food jail, to eat like normal human beings and keep their bodies at healthy weights. They don't have to eat less, they have to eat better—more often and higher-quality food. Reckless eating is not something famine sensitives can afford to do, or they will quickly end up warring with their bodies one way or another. Just like diabetics, famine-sensitive people with eating disturbances must make eating well and eating whenever they are hungry top priorities.

You can measure your famine sensitivity. Finding out how sensitive your body is to the food supply will help you understand it better so you can get well. It's not hard to do. Just take this test. Score yourself for biological relatives only and choose the number that applies most of the time.

Determining Your Famine Sensitivity

Keep a tally of the numbers that correspond to the answers you choose.

1. My personal weight history is best described as
    (0) underweight to normal weight.
    (1) slight weight problem (less than 10 pounds).
    (2) moderate weight problem (10 to 30 pounds).
    (3) very overweight (30 to 75 pounds).
    (4) morbidly obese (over 75 pounds overweight).
2. My mother is/was
    (0) underweight or normal weight.
    (1) moderately overweight (10 to 30 pounds).
    (2) very overweight (30 to 75 pounds).
    (3) morbidly obese (double normal weight).

3. My father is/was
   (0) underweight or normal weight.
   (1) moderately overweight.
   (2) very overweight.
   (3) morbidly obese.
4. What percentage of children in your family of origin (your brothers and sisters) have weight problems? Include yourself in the percentage.
   (0) No children have weight problems.
   (1) one in four or less.
   (2) one in three to one-half.
   (3) three out of four.
   (4) All children in my family have weight problems (or, if I am an only child, both of my parents and I have weight problems).
5. What percentage of your biological aunts and uncles (your mother's and father's siblings) have weight problems?
   (0) 0 to 25 percent (none to one in four).
   (1) 33 to 50 percent (one in three to one-half).
   (2) 66 to 100 percent (two in three to all).

Now add up your score. If your total falls below 3, your inherited famine sensitivity is low. This means that your body is more likely to react moderately to shortages in the food supply by the adaptive responses just described.

If you scored between 4 and 6, your famine sensitivity is moderate, or average. This means your body's tendency to react adaptively to undereating is significant. Most people fit into this category.

If your score is 7 or higher, you have high famine sensitivity. Your body is likely to be extremely tuned in to the food supply and to react powerfully to shortages of food and poor food quality. You will have to learn to eat better (not less) than most people to normalize your relationship with food.

We'll be talking more specifically about famine sensitivity in the next few chapters, but first let's take a look at the pattern that holds eating disturbances together—the Feast or Famine Cycle.

CHAPTER 3

Feast or Famine:
The Vicious Cycle
Behind Eating
Problems

A METHOD IN THE MADNESS

The symptoms associated with eating disorders follow definite patterns, which are helpful to study because the confusing symptoms of eating disturbances make a lot more sense when you look at them in relationship to one another. And recognizing these relationships can speed your progress toward normal eating. In fact, I've found that understanding these patterns is critical for anyone who is trapped in an eating disturbance and wants to be free.

The term "eating disorder" usually conjures up visions of emaciated girls working out at the local health club, their frail, overworked, skeletal frames sending shivers of aversion through most people who notice them. But people with eating disturbances come in all shapes and sizes. In fact, most are overweight. Few realize that they suffer from definite eating disturbances because most dieters learn to accept their abnormal eating patterns as normal for them—symptoms of their defective appetites, bodies and psyches. And many individuals with eating problems appear to be perfectly normal, at least weight-wise.

Regardless of body size and peculiar type of eating struggle, the underlying root of all eating disturbances is the same—undereating. Consequently, there is one fundamental pattern of eating disturbance that flows from this common cause. This pattern is a *cycle* that applies to compulsive overeating, food addiction, and bulimia which does not involve purging. Bulimia with purging and anorexia will be discussed later as shortened variations of this cycle.

I call the cycle associated with eating disorders and weight control problems the Feast or Famine Cycle. This Cycle, or some variation of it, illustrates the universal pattern experienced by people with eating problems and pathological relationships with food. It also applies to dieters and informal undereaters, regardless of the degree of their eating disturbance. Whether symptoms are mild or severe, the patterns are the same. "Successful" dieters, who usually have symptoms of bulimarexia, report that the Cycle definitely applies to them. They are just lucky enough to be able to manage their weight within a normal range. But no weight group is immune to the misery that accompanies the Cycle and its variations.

Marilyn was a chubby kid and her mom was a very chubby adult. A twenty-year veteran dieter, Marilyn's mom was so fearful of her daughter's becoming fatter and fatter as she grew up that she took her to a diet doctor when Marilyn was only nine. This doctor prescribed diet pills (amphetamines) to help little Marilyn lose weight.

Over the summer Marilyn lost twenty-five pounds—a bit more than she "needed" to lose, and a serious weight loss for a child with such a small frame. Her body was transformed and her mother was elated. But when Marilyn went back to school in the fall, she had to stop taking the diet pills. The doctor said they were only a temporary help because they were addictive.

Marilyn started gaining weight within two weeks, and by the end of the school year she had gained thirty-five pounds. Marilyn's mom begged the diet doctor to give her daughter more diet pills to reverse the trend, but he said he couldn't. He told her that Marilyn was gaining weight because she wasn't sticking with the low-calorie diet he suggested. That was true, but it wasn't the whole story.

Marilyn continued to diet off and on throughout grade school. Her mother took her to Weight Watchers with her every week for about a year. Marilyn learned to weigh her food and measure her portions. "Weighing in" at the meetings was always nerve wracking. Sometimes she did lose weight, but when she gained she was mortified. She never reached her "goal" with Weight Watchers, even though she put enormous effort and time into her diet. She knew she was cheating at times, but she got so terribly hungry. Her lack of control left Marilyn feeling like a complete failure. Her weight gradually went up because the weight she had lost, and usually a bit more, always reappeared. Once, Marilyn overheard a lifetime member (a person who reached her goal weight at one time) "whisper" to her friend as she pointed at Marilyn, "If I had been that fat as a kid, I'd have locked myself in a closet and swallowed the key." After that Marilyn refused to go.

But Marilyn's mother didn't give up. She took her discouraged daughter to her new church diet-group a few months later. Motivated by the encouragement of the group members and afraid to fail again, Marilyn lost thirty pounds over the next five months. She was terrified of having her weight gain announced to the whole group—a fear that kept her from eating anything not on her diet, for a while anyway. When she knew the weight was coming back, her group attendance ended. By the time she leveled off again, she'd gained back forty-five pounds.

Between formal diet programs Marilyn often skipped lunches because she was too embarrassed to eat in front of her classmates. She exercised, too, instead of eating breakfast, and she tried other diet tactics, such as eating only fruit on weekends or cutting out whole food groups, like starches. And of course, she overate between her diet efforts. By the tenth grade, Marilyn was 100 pounds overweight.

The Feast or Famine Cycle keeps the $30-billion diet industry well fed because diet companies charge hopeful dieters a lot of money for programmed famines. And famines do not cure weight problems or imagined weight problems; they promote weight gain and cause disturbed eating behavior. The diet industry is unique in that its methods actually worsen the problem they claim to be able to cure (as well as causing a host of other complications), thereby ensuring that clients like Marilyn will always have to return for more "help." Unfortunately, diet companies do not offer programs for the multitudes who develop eating disorders as a result of their eating-avoidance training.

It is estimated that an individual who is overweight in the United States (and countless people who are not overweight at all) will try at least two different diet methods a year in an effort to lose weight. But will they ever get thin permanently? It's extremely unlikely. Only about 10 percent of dieters are even able to stay with a program to the end, but that's not the most disturbing statistic. Over 95 percent of all dieters, no matter what method they use or how "successful" they may be at first, will gain back the weight they lose within five years of the diet, and most within two years. Nearly half of these begin a new diet even before they regain all the weight they lost.

But why? What is going on?

THE FEAST OR FAMINE CYCLE

This basic version of the Feast or Famine Cycle illustrates the eating patterns for compulsive overeaters, food addicts and bulimics who don't purge, as well as dieters whose eating disturbance is more mild. Since all individuals in these groups diet or undereat, they'll be referred to collectively as dieters, just for simplicity.

Technically, the Feast or Famine Cycle has been misnamed.It should be called the Famine or Feast Cycle because the famine is the trigger for the problem eating patterns that follow, including the feasting. The famine comes first. This is an important fact because we have been taught the exact opposite for decades. We have learned that overeating or feasting is the main problem in eating and weight struggles. So we have spent fifty years trying to fix the feasting, trying to get people to eat less, to control their eating, to stop overeating. But we haven't been very successful because the feasts don't happen all by themselves; they're triggered by the famines. The famines come first and it's the famines that must be fixed to stop the Cycle. The feasts, I have found, stop quietly as a result.

THE FEAST OR FAMINE CYCLE

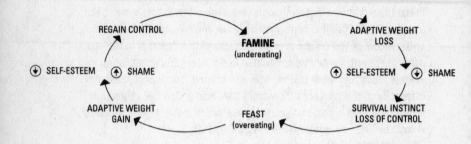

THE FIRST FAMINE

The Feast or Famine Cycle begins with the first conscious attempt to control food intake as a result of a (usually minor) weight problem. A minor weight problem can develop simply from reckless eating habits—delayed meals, skipped meals, poor-quality food, etc. Sometimes there is no extra weight at all, but only unrealistic weight standards and body-image distortion that cause people to undereat for the first time. (It's easy to get a distorted body image if you are female and living in the United States.)

This seems reasonable enough, right? If you want to lose weight, you have to try to eat less. Everybody knows that. Even a first grader in our country knows that too much food is the problem for fat people. They have to get away from food so they won't be fat anymore. So if you develop a little extra padding, get ahold of yourself, limit your intake, control your appetite. You can do it!

The only trouble is, it doesn't work in the long run because it isn't true. Often the Feast or Famine Cycle begins for a woman during puberty, when her hormones are orchestrating changes that will result in a more rounded body shape, while the culture is imprinting its very thin standard upon her. This time period, between twelve and eighteen, is when most cases of anorexia develop, and it's no coincidence. Statistics show that 50 percent of fifteen-year-old girls in the United States have already been on a diet, although less than 10 percent of them have even a minor weight problem. For at least 40 percent of these young dieters, there is no objective weight problem at all, so they don't have very far to go to become anorectic.

Others who do not diet during puberty may start undereating efforts when their lean teenage figures develop normal female curves in their twenties or thirties. These women have cultural standard problems, not weight problems. Another Cycle starter for women is childbirth. The normal weight gained during pregnancy can cause panic, even in "natural thins," that often leads to the first dieting attempts. These late-start undereaters are less likely to develop anorexia, but they are just as vulnerable to other eating disturbances.

The Feast or Famine Cycle typically catches males in their thirties and forties, although there are some important exceptions. Some men with lifelong weight problems have diet histories just like Marilyn's. They have been on the Cycle since they were children, losing and gaining in a relentless pattern. Others got into weight control as teenagers on a sports team, like wrestling, that requires boys to "make weight" in order to compete. The starving and sweating and spitting that these kids do for the sake of competing at a lower than normal weight lead some vulnerable teens right into anorexia. Bulimic purging, which enables some avoidance of weight gain from bingeing, is another dangerous tool for these young athletes. The more famine-sensitive ones simply put on excess weight after the sport season is over.

For older boys and men who don't diet, work schedules and a lack of food availability away from home frequently cause the undereating that gets them started on the Cycle.

This brings up an important fact. The starting point of the Feast or Famine Cycle, or first famine, doesn't have to be a diet. Many factors interfere with a body's ability to get enough food throughout the day, including busy schedules and subconscious food avoidance. Our culture does not prioritize our bodies' physical needs. Just the opposite is true. Our eating has to be fit into our work, school and social schedules. We eat when our breaks are allowed; we don't take breaks when we need to eat. And even if we could eat anytime, so many of us are programmed to avoid food that we probably wouldn't eat enough good food even if we could.

Anything that mimics a famine, that interferes with our eating enough quality food when we need it, can get the Feast or Famine Cycle started. This includes illness, surgery, stress (grief, financial problems, divorce, career, etc.) and medication that suppresses the appetite. Undereating, from any cause, is interpreted by the body as a famine, and so the Cycle begins.

WEIGHT LOSS—YESSSSS!

Undereating, or famining, forces the body to use fat and muscle tissue for its fuel needs to compensate for the inadequate food supply. On a typical diet about 25 percent of weight loss comes from muscle tissue, 75 percent from fat. There is always some water loss, too. Some liquid diets cause much more muscle tissue loss, and less fat, a problem that makes them quite dangerous. But dieters aren't thinking about dangerous; they're thinking about pounds and how many they can lose in the shortest amount of time.

Leave the details up to the scientists—the whole heart and soul of a dieter is focused on this one fact: you diet, you lose weight. The dieter usually doesn't care what kind of weight is being lost, just as long as that little needle moves down. And it happens. This is very, very reinforcing. The diet becomes associated with losing weight and all the wonderful things that go with being thinner: improved self-esteem, relief from guilt and shame, lifting of depression, hope for a better love life, more social acceptance and attention. Why, losing weight is just about as close as you're ever going to get to a magic potion!

People continue to diet in spite of its pitiful long-term failure rate because the weight loss associated with dieting is so exhilarating for people who desperately want to weigh less. Even temporary weight loss is extremely rewarding to people who are, or just think they are, overweight. They feel better about themselves, more secure and happy, more confident and worthy when they are losing weight. Many of the negative consequences of being overweight in our thinness-crazed culture are lessened when people lose weight. It's as if, by dieting, they're saying, "OK, I know I've got this problem, but I'm really working on it, OK?" The diet takes them off the hook somehow and gives them some sense of control—for a while. This is another key reinforcement.

Psychologically, dieting can also be used by people who feel guilty about their weight problems and want to punish themselves and their bodies. I remember doing this. And since going without food when you're hungry causes pain, it can be used as a form of self-punishment. This pain can temporarily relieve the guilt many obese people experience. (More on the reinforcements of dieting in Chapter 4.)

DENIAL

Even though the ex-dieters I have coached usually have lived miserably through decades of unsuccessful dieting, most of them, right up to the time they learned about the Feast or Famine Cycle, kept trying to diet! This is amazing when you consider the pain, expense and inconvenience of dieting. But it is true, and reflects the remarkable determination of human beings to overcome a problem in spite of repeated failures.

What makes it possible for dieters to continue to try a method that has failed them time after time *for years?* Denial.

Dieters all keep the facts about their diet experiences from sinking into their rational minds. Of course, this phenomenon is helped along by the dozens of national diet companies touting new and improved diets that the dieters haven't tried yet. But it's the psychological defense known as denial that makes those diet companies' alluring messages believable. Denial makes it possible not to see something that is blatantly obvious to others.

Just what is it that dieters have to deny in order to keep trying to lose weight by dieting? Well, it seems that they have to deny that the weight loss never lasts. But they must know that since that's the reason they keep needing another diet. What else? What are dieters unable to see that keeps them trying new diets over and over again?

LOSS OF CONTROL—
OH, NO. NO. NO. STOP. HELP!

The failing dieter must deny the fact that she always loses control of her eating behavior at some point in her diet. And she must take the blame for this loss of control and deny that the diet is faulty.

During the more than fifteen years I dieted I lost control hundreds of times, but I kept on trying new and different ways of undereating, thinking, This time will be different. This time it'll work. This diet is different. This time I'm really motivated. This time I'll keep that control all the way and then stay in control *forever.*

But it never happens that way. The dieter always loses control at some point, and when she does, the diet goes to waste. But that's not all.

Although she is blaming herself for it, this loss of control over eating behavior is her body's manifestation of its survival mechanisms at work. The famine threat has finally triggered a necessary takeover, since food really is available, and her body usurps the control of food intake. This shows up as a feast: overeating or bingeing, eating from nonhunger cues, cravings for rich foods, all to counterbalance the famine. The *diet* (or undereating effort) is the real culprit, but the rebounding dieter doesn't have a clue.

THE FEAST

Post-famine eating is typically urgent, excessive and certainly fat-producing. Normal, moderate eating is not possible for the post-famine dieter to maintain, once the loss of control occurs. Cravings are powerful and target foods from the "forbidden" list of most diets. The dieter may intermittently regain some control of her eating, but these periods are usually short-lived and are never enough to curtail the body's ultimate goal: protective fat accumulation.

Oddly, dieters out of control seldom really question this experience. Many theorize about its cause and offer such explanations as poor willpower, old eating habits, a defective appetite or body, emotional needs, stress, addiction problems, and fear of thinness resulting from psychological issues. They may think some definable force has caused their symptoms, but always deep down, they blame themselves. In fact, they have no idea what's really happening inside their bodies or the ironic role that their undereating habits play in causing their eating problems.

THE REBOUND

In its composition, weight regained is a bit different from weight lost. For example, although 25 percent of the weight lost through forced undereating is muscle tissue, there is no muscle tissue gained back. Twenty-five percent muscle lost, 0 percent regained. And that 75 percent fat loss jumps to nearly 100 percent fat when weight is regained. One hundred percent of weight that dieters gain back is fat. This means that dieters add significantly to their body fat percentage on the Feast or Famine Cycle, even if they don't gain back any more weight than they lose. Of course, undereating creates the physiological need to store more fat. Not more muscle—more fat.

The body must accomplish the task of building up the fat reserves before the next famine occurs. How long is a skinny body going to last without plenty of fat to fall back on? What if the next famine is even more severe? And for dedicated undereaters, it probably will be.

Along with regaining lost weight, dieters retrieve some old familiar feelings: battered self-esteem, shame and self-rejection. Some make vows never to put themselves through the ordeal again, the pain and disappointment are so great and the rewards so costly and fleeting. But time anesthetizes the memory, and most dieters return to undereating in some form. What else is there to do? So far, dieting has been the only option for people who want to be thinner. So even though it is a notoriously ineffective and frustrating approach, just about everyone goes back to it.

Well, that's the Feast or Famine Cycle. You're on it if you're a compulsive overeater, a so-called foodaholic or a bulimic who doesn't purge. There are really no significant differences in the Cycle patterns or the symptoms for these three groups. This is why I don't differentiate among people who use these labels—they really all have the same eating disturbance.

Bonnie had been naturally thin throughout high school and college. She started her first diet after she moved to New York City and felt overweight compared to her co-workers.

When she lost ten pounds on the Scarsdale Diet, Bonnie got a lot of compliments from friends about her new look. She also began to make occasional trips to the local deli at night for little treats. But most of the time Bonnie stuck pretty close to her diet guidelines, and she maintained her weight loss for nearly four months. She felt more confident and got plenty of kudos for her efforts, so the battle she fought with her hunger was definitely worth it.

Then something snapped. Bonnie went on a ski trip with some friends and her diet was completely derailed. The intensity of her hunger was almost shocking as Bonnie found herself overeating sometime almost every day. She reassured herself with the thought that it was just the trip and vowed to get back on the Scarsdale Diet when she got home. But she couldn't do it. Back in the city she began to give in to her cravings for ice cream at night, nearly every night. Bonnie tried compensating for these pint-sized indulgences by cutting down on lunch. But her cravings for ice cream continued to overwhelm her. She was overeating at supper more often and started feeling afraid of her own appetite, uncertain whether it could be satisfied. Bonnie was eating even after she felt full and whenever she was upset. She just couldn't seem to get ahold of herself.

Bonnie knew she was gaining weight, and she desperately tried to get back in control of her eating, but she simply couldn't. The following six months she gained sixteen pounds and finally joined Jenny Craig. Bonnie was on the Cycle.

Are You on the Feast or Famine Cycle?

Check any symptom of the Feast or Famine Cycle that applies to you:

___ 1. regular overeating and/or bingeing

___ 2. preoccupation with food and/or eating

___ 3. frequent cravings for sweets and/or high-fat foods

___ 4. eating without real hunger, especially at night

___ 5. eating in response to emotional cues or stress

___ 6. special occasion overeating

___ 7. fear and/or guilt about eating

___ 8. excessive hunger or symptoms of low blood sugar (headache, faintness, irritability, anxiety, confusion)

If you have even one symptom, you may be on the Feast or Famine Cycle. How often and how continually you are on the Cycle depends on how consistently you are undereating. If you are an occasional dieter or only rarely miss meals because you're too busy, perhaps these symptoms are not a part of your daily life. But if you are like most undereaters, this list is as familiar as the morning paper: your undereating efforts are chronically triggering your body's survival responses, causing appetite changes, make-up eating and fat storage. Remember, these symptoms are reflections of your body's need to maintain and replenish fat stores.

Some undereaters cycle several times a day, eating nothing or limiting portions at one meal, only to find themselves overeating at the next. Some cycle daily, dieting "successfully" during the day and losing control at night. Other eating-avoidant people have a three-day or weekly cycle before make-up eating takes over. And there are some dieters who can stay in control of their eating for much longer periods, like several months or even a year. The cycle varies in length, even at different times in the same person, but the patterns of undereating and overeating, weight loss and weight gain, emotional effects and loss of control are all the same.

People with eating problems are all on the Feast or Famine Cycle, or a variation of it. The symptoms of eating disturbances and the symptoms of the Feast or Famine Cycle are strikingly similar because it is the famine experience of the Cycle that sets into motion all the adaptive symptoms that we identify as eating disturbances. The Feast or Famine Cycle illustration shows the cause/effect patterns between the symptoms of eating disturbances.

A four-year veteran of Overeaters Anonymous (OA), Rita had logged thirty-one years as a dieter. She was a very successful dieter, too, and figured over the years she had lost close to a thousand pounds. But she was a maintenance failure and had gained back closer to 1,100. Ironically, Rita longed for years to just get back to the size she was when she started dieting. Now, at forty-six, she didn't even hope to get thin anymore. She just wanted some peace with food and with her body.

OA had become Rita's refuge—her only real safe place emotionally. OA members had in common a powerlessness over food, and Rita could definitely relate to that. And it was comforting to learn that others shared her problem with uncontrollable eating, experiencing the same upsetting bingeing that she did. She soon identified with the label "compulsive overeater," and oddly, it helped at least to call it something. OA didn't encourage dieting, but suggested some form of "abstinence," which each member designed for herself. Rita's was simple: no sugar, no white flour, no high-fat foods and no food between meals. This was a very uncomplicated and rather moderate plan compared to her days with Diet Center, TOPS, Nutri/System and a whole array of over-the-counter diet plans. No calorie counting, no food weighing, no food group restrictions, no pressure to lose weight or eat less than she wanted. The main problem was, it didn't help.

Rita had oatmeal and juice for breakfast, with skim milk and black coffee, usually about seven-fifteen, when she got up. She always drank a noncaloric beverage at about ten. Then she ate a whole sandwich with tuna or chicken, with low-fat mayonnaise, and a piece of fruit or a salad for lunch, around twelve-thirty. So far, so good. Another drink at three. Supper usually included a low-fat frozen dinner of pasta or chicken and vegetables, and some sugar-free frozen yogurt. It seemed like a reasonable enough plan to Rita. She weighed almost 260, so she thought she was being rather liberal with herself.

Rita's abstinence plan didn't work because, sooner or later, she always ended up bingeing, usually on foods that were on her abstinence list. For four years Rita figured, that her compulsion to overeat, an inherent defect that she couldn't control, was the cause of her bingeing. So Overeaters Anonymous gave her the support she desperately needed to weather the frustration and discouragement of living with her "compulsion." Rita would never have suspected her real problem in a million years: she wasn't eating enough.

THE BLIND LEADING THE BLIND

People on the Feast or Famine Cycle have exaggerated appetites that cannot be satisfied with "normal" amounts of food, so what would be adequate eating for a non-Cycler is undereating for Cyclers. This is one of the reasons Rita always ended up overeating. Her excessive adapted appetite never really got satisfied. Also, very heavy people sometimes require more food than lighter weights because of the extra energy they spend in just moving around. Rita's diet was far below her caloric needs because of this, too. And most obese people have distorted notions of what normal food intake is like, because of years of exposure to diet propaganda, so even when they are not dieting, they undereat. This was also a problem for Rita.

I've also observed that dieters universally experience difficulty in sensing their hunger or their fullness. This fact made it possible for Rita to tolerate her undereating for the periods that she did, but her body wouldn't adjust indefinitely. It also accounts for her ability to binge with little discomfort. These tendencies reflect Rita's adaptations to the intermittent famines of dieting.

Besides disturbed eating, the net results of the Feast or Famine Cycle are cyclic weight loss and gain that usually adds pounds over the years, plus the stress and misery that inevitably accompany these weight and eating fluctuations. Recently, some research studies have suggested that there may be some potentially serious long-term physical consequences of weight cycling, including increased vulnerability to diabetes, heart disease and even premature death. But whether or not it's a sure thing that yo-yo dieting has serious physical consequences, the emotional turmoil that it invariably puts people through should be enough to justify strongly cautioning people against it.

CYCLE AWARENESS AND EMOTIONS

When undereaters who suffer from distorted eating patterns finally learn about the Feast or Famine Cycle, they are always relieved. They realize that the shame, guilt and blame they have suffered are really misplaced. They finally understand how truly powerless they have been to solve their eating and weight problems in a lasting way. They also discover how ironic it is that their efforts to stay slim or lose weight have inadvertently kept them locked in food jail, and sometimes overweight besides. Many recovering ex-dieters say they feel they have been released from jail by this information. But relief isn't the only feeling they have.

Ex-dieters who find out the facts about the Feast or Famine Cycle are angry, too. And they are sad. They have lost so much—time, energy, money. Some have suffered serious setbacks—marriage, health, career. Led down a dead end, dieters have been set up for failure.

When weight-conscious undereaters see their own patterns in the Feast or Famine Cycle, sooner or later they remember the diet doctor who put them on diet pills when they were just nine years old. Or they recall the diet group leader who embarrassed them in front of their friends, or the nurse in that "medically supervised" program who accused them of cheating on 800 calories a day. Yet they weren't cheating—they were starving and irritable and weak and nervous and weepy and without energy, but, by God, they weren't cheating. And they remember the rejection, the looks, the loneliness, the endless struggle, the prejudice. They recall the eating disorders specialist who said they'd never be well unless they learned to bare their souls in group. And they remember the sermon about gluttony. They remember the never-ending longing to have a normal appetite and a normal body—just to be able to eat without worrying about it all the time. And they remember the labels: compulsive overeater, food addict, emotional binger, freak, pig. No wonder they are sad and angry.

POWER

People who have been victimized have to get over it if they want to get on with productive and successful lives. Nearly all of us have, at one time or another, experienced victimization. The difference between the people who are no longer victims and those who are still victims is the experience of empowerment. Why wouldn't everybody choose to become empowered? Because powerful people learn to accept responsibility and solve problems instead of blaming others. And blaming others is much easier than accepting responsibility and solving problems.

If you want to have a normal relationship with food, but you just can't see giving up blaming other people or organizations, and you don't want all that much responsibility or work, then you're only dreaming. It will never happen for a victim. It takes too much courage, determination and power.

VARIATIONS ON THE FEAST OR FAMINE CYCLE

Two groups of eating disorders don't fit the complete Cycle pattern because they involve behaviors that interfere with the completion of the Cycle as it has just been illustrated. These two groups are bulimics who purge and anorectics who do not lose control of their restrictive eating patterns. Let's take a look at bulimic purging and its effect on the Cycle pattern.

THE FEAFAM CYCLE OF BULIMIA

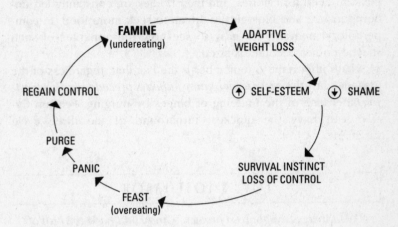

Bulimics who use purging to get rid of food they eat during a binge have discovered a deadly way of "beating" the weight gain produced by the adaptations of the Feast or Famine Cycle. Although purging usually seems quite innocent and benign when a person first tries it, in time, the bulimic binge/purge cycle exacts a high toll both emotionally and physically. Bulimics are especially trapped in their self-destructive eating patterns because they think they have found the key to escaping the weight gain caused by bingeing. But purging is no emancipator. It actually locks them into food jail with a dangerous combination of fear and delusions of control.

In order to short-circuit the Cycle before weight gain occurs as a result of bingeing or overeating, bulimics get rid of the food they eat during the loss of control phase, mainly by vomiting. Food that gets through to the intestinal tract can be flushed out with laxatives. Any calories that might have been absorbed quickly through the stomach can be worked off in aerobic exercise, before they are stored as fat. The bulimic Cycle is called the FeaFam because its distinctive feature is the aborted feast. Purging dramatically interferes with the body's struggle for make-up food, creating physiological conflict and confusion unparalleled in other eating problems.

Purging is a feature unique to bulimia because the vomiting makes it possible to get back to the famine much sooner than Cyclers who feast and allow their bodies to digest and use the food. It also accounts for the tremendous preoccupation and obsession with food that these purgers report. Their feasts never satisfy their physical need for calories, and their bodies are constantly left undernourished and biologically driven to seek more food, in compensatory amounts. It's easy to see how the appetites of such starved bodies become ox-sized.

What's important to remember is the fact that, regardless of the Cycle length, *famines (undereating) always precede binges (feasting)*. Because of the undoing of binges by purging, FeaFam Cyclers can have the quickest turnaround of the three cycle variations.

LOVE'S LOST LABOR

Mildly overweight as a preteen, Cindy had been the butt of some cruel jokes and comments during junior high that left her especially sensitive about her body shape. Although she lost most of her extra padding during the first two years of high school, Cindy still took her few extra pounds very seriously. She wanted to get slim like her lankier friends, so she started dieting the summer before her junior year. She wasn't much of an athlete, but she forced herself to jog three miles a day. The weight came off. Then Cindy met Mark.

A college student home working for the summer, Mark was far too handsome and athletic for Cindy, or so she thought. They met at the high school track when both of them were running. He smiled. She was embarrassed. He started a conversation. She stumbled over her words. He wanted to know, could he see her again sometime? This was frightening and exciting for Cindy, who hadn't received much attention from boys.

When they started dating Cindy's weight became paramount to her. She couldn't be fat and date an athlete, especially a gorgeous athlete. She "knew" he would never have looked at her before she lost weight, so controlling her eating was now her number-one priority—after Mark. Even though she had lost over ten pounds and looked thin, Cindy adopted the adage, "You can never be too rich or too thin." She figured she'd probably never be that rich, but she was going to be thin—really thin—drop-dead gorgeous thin.

Cindy continued the same diet she had found in a magazine, limiting her calories to 800 a day and running every day. It had been responsible for her weight loss before she met Mark, and now it was going to make her even more feminine and attractive, and as far away from the plump days of eighth grade as she could get. Occasionally, Cindy would overindulge, but she just added miles to her running to compensate. But then something happened that refocused her whole world, something Cindy wouldn't have imagined in a million years.

While she was house-sitting for a friend one weekend, Cindy combed the cupboards for something to eat. She was absolutely starving. Tortilla chips—too fatty, too many calories. Old brownies with frosting—way too rich. Carrot juice, yep. Veggies for a salad, yep. Water-packed tuna in a can, OK. But after eating, Cindy went back to the kitchen. Back to the brownies. Oh, just one little piece. I haven't had chocolate in ages, she thought.

Twenty-five minutes later Cindy had finished half a pan of old brownies, the whole bag of tortilla chips, a box of macaroon cookies, a quart of seafood pasta salad, two frozen cheese danish pastries and nearly a half gallon of chocolate chip ice cream. She was numb as she ate in a mechanical way. She didn't really taste anything. She hardly chewed the food before she gulped it down like a desperate animal. The reality or consequences of what she was doing didn't surface to her conscious until she had just about finished the ice cream. Then terror struck.

Cindy felt sick. She felt as if her stomach would explode. She didn't know how long she had been eating. It was like waking up from a nightmare, only it wasn't over. She couldn't let this food get to her body. Instinctively, she headed for the bathroom.

Afterward she told herself it was an emergency, she'd never do it again. She would stay in control next time.

Only two days later the next time came, and Cindy

couldn't stay in control. She was shocked. Well, two emergencies don't make an eating disorder. But two or three or four "emergencies" a day for eight years do.

In spite of her purging and constant effort to control her eating, Cindy gained back the ten pounds she'd lost that summer. And she lost the boyfriend she'd gained. No one will ever convince Cindy that the two facts weren't related.

Other facts that Cindy needed to connect were her strict diet/exercise periods and her bingeing. Her wild eating episodes simply triggered the potent fear of weight gain, and that set off Cindy's only effective solution—purging. All these relationships eluded Cindy, who finally went for help at an eating disorders clinic after three years of FeaFam cycling. There they told her that her bulimia was a result of her broken relationship with Mark (which happened after her bulimia developed) and suppressed anger at her parents.

Are You on the FeaFam Cycle?

Check out these symptoms of the FeaFam Cycle to see if you fit this food jail pattern:

_____ 1. strict dieting or efforts to control food intake, with or without drug aids

_____ 2. excessive appetite

_____ 3. loss of control over eating behavior

_____ 4. overeating or bingeing

_____ 5. purging or wasting of food by self-induced vomiting, laxative and/or diuretic abuse, and/or exercise

_____ 6. high anxiety about weight gain and eating

_____ 7. distorted body image

_____ 8. preoccupation with eating and weight

FeaFam Cyclers are very likely to have every symptom listed, in addition to the physical effects of the Cycle that we talked about earlier. If you don't, but you can identify at least numbers 1, 4, and 5, then this Cycle variation is a fit for you.

THE FAMINE TRACK OF ANOREXIA

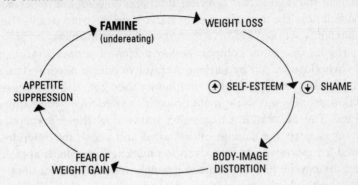

The third variation on the Feast or Famine Cycle is called the Famine Track because, for true anorexia, no feasting is involved, and because it is so short, "track" is a more accurate term than "cycle." The Famine Track involves only the first third of the Feast or Famine Cycle: famine in the form of controlled undereating, resulting weight loss, reinforcements of weight loss, body-image distortion and consequent fear, and back to famine. This is the least complicated and usually most dangerous pattern of disturbed eating. It is the picture of an anorectic—a person set in a deadly conflict against the instincts of her own body.

The eating pattern for anorexia is pretty simple on the surface. Anorectics just constantly undereat, right? Yes, but there's a bit more to it than that. In order to "just constantly undereat," people on the Famine Track must continuously overcome their bodies' survival instincts regarding food. They must willfully and successfully overcome their urge to eat, creating self-imposed chronic starvation. All of the adaptive appetite changes that go with famine survival must be submitted to the will of the anorectic.

In order to keep their adapting bodies and threatening appetites under control, anorectics must keep quite an arsenal of weapons and strategies ready. Anorectics are not just passively undereating; they are deliberately, forcefully, actively, purposefully and conscientiously controlling their intake of food. They have to. If they let their guard down, they know they'd certainly lose control and start eating more.

On the Famine Track, anorectics overcome their bodies' mechanisms for taking over the eating controls to prevent starvation. How do they do it? As far as I can tell, by sheer determination at first, and later on, probably by virtue of the brain chemistry imbalance of starvation. This determination and consequent imbalance make it possible for anorectics to starve themselves to death. They sometimes actually win over their own survival instincts.

There's one other complicating symptom of anorexia. Anorectics who lose weight by starving themselves almost never feel thin. In fact, they often feel fatter the thinner they get. This strange reaction propels the Cycle that anorectics experience—the Famine Track. The illustration on page 75 shows how these perceptual changes keep the famine efforts alive and cause the relentless need for more weight loss, even in emaciated people. It appears that the psyche fills in the missing weight rebound part of the Cycle by altering the perception of body weight in the absence of real feasting.

THE FEAR FACTOR

Anorectics sometimes suffer from a lack of appetite, which reflects one way the body adapts to low food availability. In my experience, though, most anorectics *do* feel hunger at times, but always with fear. Actually, fear and anxiety usually *suppress* the appetite in normal people because of the fight or flight response—to keep the digestive tract shut down in order to prepare for danger. This could explain why anorectics, who universally suffer from a phobia of weight gain (which they associate with eating anything), can consistently ignore hunger, aided by their fear and its physical effect on their appetite.

Anorectics' appetites sometimes become enormous, which is reflected in their losing control and crossing over to the FeaFam Cycle. Their intense fear of weight gain, coupled with their adapted monster appetites, which also provoke fear, leaves anorectics without much choice but to maintain control, or die, some of them say. And control at the absolutely thinnest weight possible adds some insurance against the possibility of ever losing their grip on that huge appetite lurking within.

At fifteen, Bridget started dieting with two of her girlfriends, just to see if they could lose weight. None of the three had a weight problem, they just wanted to see what the diet hoopla was all about. Bridget lost two pounds the first week, which made her feel like a success. Her friends didn't lose anything, so they decided to give their experiment another week or two. Bridget lost five more pounds the following weeks and started to enjoy her clothes loosening up and her more dramatic cheekbones. Her friends gave the diet up—it was too much work and they got too hungry. But Bridget was hooked.

Twenty pounds and eight weeks later, Bridget's friends finally told her she was too thin. She looked at them with real surprise. "Too thin?! You sound like my mom," she replied. "My stomach is huge. I have to take off at least five more pounds just to get my stomach down to normal." This was the first time her friends had ever heard Bridget complain about her body. It wouldn't be the last.

Bridget was hospitalized six months later, her five-foot eight-inch frame held together by barely a hundred pounds. Over the next six years she was admitted to the eating disorders unit fifteen different times.

WHO CAN RECOVER FROM EATING DISORDERS?

The program coming up in the next chapters will be helpful and even healing for many people who are searching for answers to their eating problems. But this path for healing won't work for some people, and I'll tell you why. It's too hard for a while, and that while is too long for some. Some people aren't willing to work that hard, not even for relief from the torture of food jail. Others are too afraid of letting go, of trusting anyone or anything besides themselves. But hard work and trust are things that getting free requires, along with discipline and perseverance. Some people can't or won't exercise the discipline it takes and others lack the ability to tolerate the delay in gratification. This is not a quick and easy plan for relief from eating problems. There is no such thing. This strategy requires considerable maturity, I have found, and some people are not willing to grow up that much.

What about you? Are you ready to work? Are you willing to let go? Then roll up your sleeves and say a prayer, because we're about to take on the fiend that's been running your life. And we're going to beat it and get you set free from food jail forever.

Two

The Program for Breaking Free

CHAPTER 4

Getting Off the Cycle: Challenges in Learning to Eat Enough

BREAKING A CYCLE OF PATHOLOGICAL EATING PATTERNS is no easy task. There are many challenges for you and your body in this new approach to eating, but you are not alone. Everyone who wants to reclaim a healthy relationship with food is faced with these obstacles, and anyone who is willing to work hard and face her fears can successfully get off the Feast or Famine Cycle and its variations. It takes time, but be patient. You and your precious body are worth it.

There are two main goals that we're aiming for. The first goal is:

to stop undereating completely.

This means learning to stop dieting, and to stop overregulating the amount of food you eat and when you eat it. This is about giving up the intellectual controls for eating. So, you're probably asking, if our intellects don't control our eating, where will the control come from? This is where the second goal comes in:

to learn to eat, and to stop eating, in response to body signals alone.

I call this "body-controlled eating." It is the key to solving the loss of control problems and normalizing the gigantic appetites that people with disturbed eating experience.

I can hear your protests: Wait just a minute. You mean to tell me that we're supposed to stop controlling our food intake com-

pletely, and give up deciding how much and when to eat? And
then, you're asking us to just let our bodies control these things—
our bodies, for heaven's sake? What exactly are we after here, the
record for the all-time fastest weight gain for human beings in the
universe since time began?

No, but your concerns about letting go are legitimate and understandable. Everybody has them. They're about not trusting
your body and fearing your appetite. As an undereater, you've
learned that your body can't be trusted when it comes to eating. In
the past, as soon as you let your guard down, you've been likely
to lose control and overeat. Or, if you're anorectic, you have to
channel all your energies so that you absolutely make sure your
guard never goes down because of this likelihood.

So why would you be willing to turn eating controls over to
your body? I'll tell you: Because the reason your body has been so
crazy about food is your undereating. And once you remedy that
cause, you know it can gradually normalize and get into healthy
control. Bodies are designed to manage food intake and maintain
lean, healthy body weights. When bodies are given back the controls they are designed to have and should have kept all along, the
people they house are freed to do other things with their minds.
This is the basic premise of your escape from food jail.

At any rate, your fears are normal. Go ahead and admit them:
I'M TERRIFIED OF LETTING GO OF MY EATING CONTROLS!

There, does that feel better? A little? No? Well, just hold on while
I walk you through the process. Once you understand what you're
doing and why, and see that it's the only way, you'll probably feel
a bit less frantic.

This chapter is designed to help you negotiate your way out of
compulsive or habitual undereating as quickly and as comfortably
as possible. In Chapter 5 you will learn the directions to your second goal, the sane world of body-controlled eating.

WHY IS IT SO HARD TO STOP UNDEREATING?

Limiting your food intake and fighting your hunger are painful,
frustrating and downright depressing at times. So why should it be
so hard to stop doing these things? Those who have never struggled to control their weight by controlling their eating cannot understand the tremendous adjustment dieters have to face when

they decide to stop undereating. You'd think it would be the most natural thing in the world to stop inflicting this kind of pain on your own body, and it is natural, but it's definitely not easy. In fact, ending the diet lifestyle forever is almost always very difficult and very frightening for undereaters, but especially for those with eating disturbances. Here are some of the reasons this change is often so hard.

Remember that the Feast or Famine Cycle and its variations are perpetuated by intermittent reinforcements. Dieters get certain "payoffs" from the diet lifestyle, for all the pain they bear in the process. And as you may recall from the last chapter, even the pain itself can serve as a payoff. The more obvious rewards that dieting can bring, including quick weight loss and improved self-esteem—both temporary perks—have been discussed. But there are more subtle reinforcers that come with dieting and undereating that can make quitting tough.

Although weight loss is the central motivator and reinforcer for dieting, other rewards develop with the undereating lifestyle. Chronic dieting provides a tremendous escape or distraction from many relatively serious challenges of life. Preoccupied dieters can maintain quite a detachment from problems that they may be afraid of or simply don't want to face, whether consciously or unconsciously.

To different degrees, the Feast or Famine Cycle and its variations can be emotionally as well as physically debilitating, promoting a victim attitude. This victim role, with its crippling self-pity, is sometimes adopted as a life script. I have observed that, in most cases, undereaters are not even aware of the escapist nature or victim aspect of their diet obsession. Dieting has simply taken over in their lives in ways they never intended, don't realize and cannot control, once the Cycle is well established.

You may also remember from the last chapter that dieters can also be reinforced by the pain of dieting itself. Many Cycling undereaters feel bad about themselves because of their weight and/or eating problems. They often feel, if only subconsciously, that they deserve to be punished simply for having those weight or eating problems, and for the obvious part they themselves play in perpetuating them.

The attitude that they must pay for their "sins" is promoted by many pervasive cultural attitudes about overweight people: they are gluttonous, they are lazy, they have no willpower, they don't care, etc. These are all common moralistic labels. Of course, the best way to pay for sins of overindulgence is to counterbalance them by underindulgence in the form of strict dieting or even fasting. For some of these "sinners," dieting is a necessary penance, and the pain that accompanies chronic or intermittent undereating serves an important emotional role. This applies to people on all variations of the Feast or Famine Cycle because they all tend to perceive these principles as relevant to themselves, at least subjectively.

GOALTENDER

One extremely subtle kickback from dieting involves goals. Many people are uncomfortable with goal-setting in their own lives. It's risky to have goals. When you set them, you risk failing. It requires a certain commitment and investment in one's own life. Goals are about who we are and what we believe in. Goal-setting is about direction-setting, which requires change, and change is a form of stress, and stress is painful. Voluntary pain goes against human nature, so people are generally disinclined to even think about their life goals, much less actually decide on some.

On the other hand, there is something in us that keeps inspiring us to change, to reach out, to explore, to do more with our lives. Call it creativity, call it desire for growth, call it human nature—it is undoubtedly there. And it creates a problem: we have an urge to improve, to change, to reach goals for ourselves despite the stress and pain involved. This conflict between our avoidant natures and our need to grow influences whether we set goals and why we set them if we do.

But here's an interesting twist. Because of our desire to improve ourselves, plus our tendency to avoid change, superficial, petty goals can interfere with our having substantial, grand goals. There is something in us that pushes us to keep growing, stretching, reaching new levels in life, but often we don't reach, stretch or grow in bigger ways when we are consumed with mundane concerns and activities. Or perhaps we choose to stay focused on goals that keep our view narrow instead of broad, goals that do not challenge the real depth of our human potential. We avoid greatness because we are afraid, and there are plenty of non-

threatening things to do to help us feel as if we're getting somewhere, like dieting.

This process is usually insidious, but obsessive food-intake
management commonly interferes with personal development. Individuals who are otherwise ambitious, creative souls too often
become engrossed in meticulous dietary restrictions and weight-
loss goals to the near exclusion of other, more valuable endeavors.
This is a tragedy. The waste of human potential can hardly be estimated, especially among women.

WHO AM I AGAIN?

*A housewife for eighteen years, Anne worked part-time as
a bank teller when her children were all in school. She was
popular with the customers and her co-workers because of
her bright smile and quick sense of humor. This position was
higher than Anne ever expected to get in the business world.
She had been dieting constantly for thirty years, and bulimic
for six.*

*About a year after Anne got off the Feast or Famine Cycle,
she told me she was a painter—oils and acrylics. I was surprised. She had gone to a school of fine art for almost three
years after high school, but dropped out because she ran out
of money, then got married and was soon busy caring for her
young family. Once dieting became her life focus, she stopped
painting and didn't really think about it until sometime after
she learned to eat again. Then her interest in art returned,
along with some long-lost confidence, and after painting for
six months she decided to do a show of her work. Two years
later she did. The following year Anne bought a small art
gallery with another artist. Anne told me it never would have
happened if she hadn't gotten her eating straightened out
first.*

Giving up the relatively superficial goals of dieting—achieving
weight loss, reaching target weight, eating according to rigid rules,
sticking with the diet, never eating certain foods, keeping a record
of every morsel of food eaten, etc.—can leave quite a void, eliminating all this structure and expectations in a person's daily rou-

tine. Giving up controlled undereating can leave a person insecure, fearful, confused and/or depressed. You'd think ending such
a torturous lifestyle would be a complete relief, but it's not, especially for those whose eating disturbances have overshadowed
much of the rest of their lives.

WHEN FOOD AVOIDANCE "WORKS"

There are people who manage to maintain normal body
weights by chronic or regular dieting efforts. We call these individuals "artificially thin." They may be quite arrogant about their bodies because they believe that if they can do it by sheer willpower
and determination, then anybody can. Usually hooked on dieting
as a way of life, people in this group tend to focus their goals on
their body shape, weight and workout schedules. But unfortunately, these "successful" dieters pay a very high price for their
thinness, and unless their goal is to be underweight the cost is
quite unnecessary.

The work that artificially thin people do to keep their bodies
trim is often considerable and there is nothing inherently wrong
with this effort. It can even be considered admirable. But it can
also become extreme and out of balance, posing a serious distraction from other important areas of life.

WHAT'S YOUR GOAL NOW?

If you just want to be thin, no matter what the cost in the short
or long run, and you don't mind giving up a goodly portion of
your future energy and your health to maintain your thinness by
hunger-control tactics and/or binge reversal methods, then the
diet/eating disturbance lifestyle may still be an option for you.
Maybe you're not ready to get out of food jail right now. You figure you have time. You're young and thin and energetic, so what's
the hurry? Am I going to try to talk you into changing? Is this book
designed to persuade you to fix your sick eating habits when they
seem to be working pretty well for you right now? No and no.

Of course, if you are already overweight from the Feast or
Famine Cycle, then you know dieting won't ever lead to your

weight goal and keep you there (you're too famine sensitive), so it looks as if the decision to stop dieting is made for you. It's not.

As you consider your personal goal, keep these facts in mind:

The system that works for people in their teens and twenties often fails to keep them svelte and healthy in their thirties and forties.

Some serious health consequences of bulimia, anorexia or bulimarexia develop only years after these disorders begin.

The cycle that caused moderate weight struggles during the second and third decades of life can lead to more significant trouble and weight gain in the fourth and fifth decades.

There are many consequences of weight cycling and long-term undereating besides living in jail. You can probably make a list of your own.

It's also worth considering the fact that getting off the Cycles is generally easier the sooner it is done, preferably before a serious weight and/or eating problem has developed.

Check below if the statement definitely applies to you:

—I want to overcome my obsessive, compulsive preoccupation with food.
—I'd like to put the pleasure back into my eating and the joy back into my exercise.
—I long to have a normal relationship with food and with my body.
—I am convinced that dieting will never accomplish and/or maintain my figure goals without disturbing my eating behavior.
—I believe that there is a better way, a more normal way to manage my eating.

If you're sure about most of these, you've come to the right place to move toward your goal.

YOU DECIDE

Whatever you are thinking about your body, your eating struggles and your future health, you have a decision to make. I'm assuming, since you're reading this book, that you are hoping to overcome the eating patterns that entrap your life. But that's not enough. You still have to make a decision, even if it's simply to keep exploring ways to get better. And perhaps some readers will not be ready to abandon their self-destructive cycle for some reason—fear of weight gain, of change, of losing control. They must make a decision, too, to continue to live in food jail.

So, what is *your* goal? It's wise to put your goal on paper. This helps you realize and absorb it better. For example, you might write:

My goal is to have a normal and healthy relationship with food and to be completely free of purging.

(signature)

(date)

My goal is to stop dieting and obsessing about my weight.

(signature)

(date)

My goal is to overcome my fear of being fat and my fear of healthful foods so I can stay at an appropriate weight.

(signature)

(date)

My goal is to develop a healthy body image so I can stop trying to get smaller than I was meant to be.

(signature)

(date)

Write your goal down, no matter what stage you're at in your plan to get well. Even a small goal, like eating more for breakfast every day, can be a place to start, but try to put your *ultimate goal* down on paper—even if it seems impossible right now. It's empowering just to say what you want to accomplish, and it also makes you realize that no one else is responsible for your eating disturbance. You're making the choices to keep it going or end it forever, now that you're finding a way out.

DIET ADDICTION: HOOKED ON UNDEREATING

Much has been written about so-called food addiction, based on the observations of many researchers, psychologists and dieters themselves who report compulsive, out-of-control eating behavior. As I said in Chapter 1, I have never observed these "addictive" eating patterns in anyone except undereaters. This is why I dismiss the term "food addict." There is no such thing, unless you want to label us all with the term and add to it "air addicted" and "water addicted." People who do not eat enough food on a regular basis tend to get compulsive about food, and eat without control at times, but this is an adaptive response, not the result of some primary addictive process. There is, however, an addictive process involved in the Cycles. It is the addiction to dieting.

An "addiction" is defined as "a behavior or relationship which cannot be given up without aid in spite of the destructive nature and negative consequences of the behavior or relationship." People with eating problems who want to stop undereating often cannot do so without support, in spite of their determination. They have anxiety and often feel powerless to overcome their compulsive urge to try to eat less food than they want and need. The greatest problem I've encountered as an eating disorders coach is compulsive undereating—the tendency people have to continue to try to control portions and eat less than they desire, even after they've been carefully taught that they must eat more in order to get off the Cycle and get well. You'd think these underfed individuals would jump at the chance to eat until they are really full, but they often don't. They are too afraid, and they are addicted to dieting.

Undereating becomes a lifestyle focus for most serious long-term weight controllers, and certainly for those who develop disturbed eating patterns. It becomes an integral part of their identity, just as a job is for many people. Besides providing a relatively innocuous topic to think and talk about, dieting can become a safe place to focus energy, friendships and social activities. Weight-conscious people can get excited about weight-control information and diet behaviors. They can also escape temporarily from the problems of real life and get emotionally high on weight loss. Even when their lives are a mess, undereaters admit that their diet success has the power to make everything much more tolerable.

Undereaters, especially anorectics, literally get high by becoming dangerously hungry, a physiological state accompanied by elevated insulin levels. Insulin has mood-altering properties. And the fat-burning that accompanies starvation produces ketones, which are also known biochemical mood elevators. These biochemical changes probably play significant roles in the development of eating disorders that involve morbid undereating. Diet addiction is clearly both psychological and biological. But the cornerstone motive to undereat remains: the cultural standard for beauty.

THE THIN IDEAL

There is enormous pressure in our culture to be thin, especially for women. Everyone knows the old saying that one cannot be too rich or too thin. The message that you're never thin enough is supported most relentlessly by our fashion trends, which flaunt extremely thin female models, especially in women's magazines. These pervasive images pressure women to diet—even those who are not the least overweight. The subtle message is malignant. It puts women, especially young developing girls who are especially concerned about their attractiveness, at risk for eating disturbances and obesity. More on these topics in Chapters 5 and 6. These attitudes and standards in our culture do more to promote the diet lifestyle and all the physical disorders and emotional pain that go with it than anything else.

GETTING OFF THE CYCLE: WITHDRAWAL

Because undereating and weight management become such a focal point in life for the eating disturbed, Cyclers usually experience some common symptoms of withdrawal when they start to eat more normally. These symptoms are related to the process of letting go of controls long and tenaciously held, and learning to take in the very thing they have worked so hard to avoid. But these withdrawal symptoms are especially connected to weight gain.

Almost all people with eating disturbances who learn about the influence that undereating has over their appetites, minds and eating behavior realize that they need to learn to eat more food if they're ever going to recover. But it's not quite that simple. Once they understand it, often panic sets in. The object of their fear, and phobia in some cases, is the remedy that they must take: food. It's hard to eat more in a panic.

Even after the initial attempts to increase food intake have calmed the panic they first feel, bulimics, anorectics and compulsive overeaters almost always continue to have chronic anxiety about food and eating for some time—even if their weights remain stable. But if they gain, panic returns like a demon and, along with it, the temptation of the safety of controlled undereating and food avoidance. They may return to the security of familiar habits. Many succumb during the first months. To borrow an AA term, this is a "slip" for the person who wants to break out of food jail. It's common and not fatal, but it warrants some action.

The eating-disturbed person in remission who returns to undereating as a way of solving her anxiety about weight gain is "slipping" back into traditional diet thinking. It's the diet propaganda that got her trapped into disturbed eating in the first place, but it's a familiar road, and comfortable in some ways. The antidote for this regression is simple. This frightened individual needs to remind herself about the facts of eating, healthy weight and appetite, and especially about the effects of undereating on her body and psyche. Reviewing this book would be helpful. Looking back over her diet and eating struggles would, too. Talking with a person who has successfully broken the Cycle could be very reassuring as well. More about support later in this chapter.

LOSS AND GRIEF

Anytime people are uprooted from habits, traditions or familiar behaviors they experience a sense of loss. This is true regardless of how healthful the changes are. We seem to become attached to our behavior patterns, for better or worse, and this is one of the chief reasons that quitting destructive behaviors is so difficult and complicated. The benefits hoped for are up against powerful negative feelings happening right now.

Giving up controlled undereating as a lifestyle is often perceived as a loss at first. This sense of loss can trigger depression or other grief symptoms. It may feel to the mending undereater that a piece of her personality has been cut away. If she doesn't understand what is happening and how to help herself, she may revert to undereating to regain her emotional bearings.

This sense of loss is typically about two areas: personal control and life focus. Personal control over food intake is a big deal to anyone with an eating disturbance. As I have suggested earlier, this control is always the starting point of eating problems, as well as the fuel that keeps them going. Maintaining controlled undereating is a goal near the heart of every person who has an eating disturbance because of long-held beliefs, long-practiced habits and long-cherished weight ideals. Consequently, giving up such revered tenets and behaviors can inspire powerful feelings of loss.

The central role that dieting or undereating assumes in the life of the eating disturbed becomes quite a problem when it is given up. There seems to be a void created by this shift, and although temporary, it can be upsetting. Ex-undereaters complain of boredom because of this void, and it usually takes some time before they can fill their lives with other productive thoughts and activities. There can also be a sense of loss, and the program outlined in the coming chapters deals specifically with this loss and the needs it provokes.

SURFACING OF EVADED ISSUES

When much of your life has been wrapped up in crazy eating behavior, possibly for years, it can be quite a shock to surface from an eating disturbance and find yourself on the face of the earth with other important things to do besides trying to get thinner. In fact, other important things sometimes present themselves rather dramatically after having been stored away while you were worried day and night about whether, when, what and how much to eat every single moment of every single day. I call this "waking up." You think your eating problems have brought troubles, just wait until you start solving those problems!

An amazing number of people who are getting over eating disorders tell me that, in the process, they discover some important but neglected areas of their lives. Some see their marital problems for the first time. Others notice troubles in their relationships with their children or parents. Quite a few start therapy to deal with old issues or to improve their emotional health. Almost all uncover interests, friends, talents or goals they had all but forgotten in the land of perpetual eating management.

The Big "If" Checkup

Pretend your body is perfect for a moment, and you can eat anything. Everything you want to wear fits. Your body is legendary—effortlessly lean and muscular. Now look at the rest of your life:

What needs more of your attention?
What interests or gifts have you been neglecting?
Do you have any long-lost goals?
Friendships to nurture?
Volunteer work to pursue?
Career change to plan for?
Rest or recreation needs you want to enjoy?
Vacation destinations to dream about?

ALL ALONE AND NEEDING SUPPORT

With the panic, anxiety, depression, loss, grief and new roster of challenges to cope with, people who are trying to get back to normal eating need support, and a lot of it. Anxiety alone provokes the urge to have someone near, someone who understands, will listen and encourage, and just be there. The particular people you choose for support will make all the difference, so choose carefully.

Because eating troubles have traditionally been approached from the psychological perspective, programs and support groups for people trying to recover have focused on psycho-emotional issues. This is a big problem for those who decide to break out of food jail because the approach presented here doesn't accept the idea that overeating is emotional, but teaches that it's physical, and that the focus of recovery from disturbed eating must be physical, too. This is a program of learning to eat, and it's good news. Since you're probably going to have emotional struggles as long as you're alive, isn't it great to know you can learn to eat normally while you're still an emotional wreck? You bet it is. (More on support later in this chapter.)

HOW TO STOP UNDEREATING: STEP ONE

For the sake of simplicity, I'm going to call this program of recovery from eating problems the Naturally Thin Program, which I introduced in my first book. This approach to eating disturbances is very different from everything else out there. This unique program shifts the blame for weight gain from eating too much to *eating avoidance* (dieting and undereating), and focuses on one goal to get eating-disturbed people out of food jail forever: *ending the famines*. This is why your first goal is to stop undereating completely. But in order to do that you need to understand how and why the famines, diets and weight-control tactics are causing the eating problems. This information, outlined in the first three chapters, gives you some incentive to begin to eat more, more often and more healthfully. Remember, *undereating is the trigger* for the adaptive responses that those with disturbed eating experience as symptoms, and until this undereating is remedied there is no hope for a lasting recovery.

In order to end your undereating habits, you'll have to, at first, ignore, and then eventually unlearn, almost everything you now know about eating for weight control. Let's first take a look at what you "know."

According to traditional diet theory, calories are bad and eating the fewest number of calories possible is therefore best for those who want to lose weight or stay thin. Since eating less is the goal of the traditional diet approach, hunger signals are often ignored or left undersatisfied. This is supposed to be necessary and perfectly benign—just a part of the price thin people have to pay. Feelings of actual fullness are to be avoided and often eating between meals is frowned upon. Diet foods are "best." Foods with any fat in them are evil. Keeping food away from hungry dieters is considered a helpful tactic. Exercise is thought necessary to burn off calories lest they most certainly be stored as fat.

See how much you've learned in your quest for thinness? Now we'll address these false diet tenets from the "breaking-out" perspective of adaptation.

DIET DOCTRINE #1: Calories are bad, so eat as few as possible.

The much-maligned calorie is really just a unit of energy, but undereaters hate calories as if they were malignant. They look for "no-calorie" and "low-calorie" foods, even if they have to pay more money for them. This is because they aren't worried about getting their money's worth in calories; they're worried about getting fat. And everybody knows, too many calories make you fat, right? Wrong.

It's just not that simple, and because of adaptation, avoiding adequate calories actually promotes eating disturbances and weight gain. This is a fact you simply must get ahold of in order to begin to eat enough, to stop undereating and perpetuating the Cycle you've been on. You need enough calories, a minimum, in order to get well, so start eating more good food when you get hungry. Quality calories are good for you. When you eat enough they keep you from craving, and bingeing on, lousy food. In fact, you want to eat the amount of high-quality calories* that your body asks for every day. (Remember, your body will tell you how much food it needs.) Then its fuel needs will be well met and your appetite can get back to normal.

Quality calories are good for you, so eat enough to satisfy your hunger every day.

DIET DOCTRINE #2: Eating the least possible food is best.

People with eating disturbances often "medicate" their hunger with as little food as they can get by with. They rarely really satisfy their hunger because they believe that doing so would lead to

---

* High-quality calories are found in all Real Foods (typical meal foods) that are low in sugar and fat. See the Real Foods list in the Appendix (pages 277–280).

weight gain. They're right in a limited way because their adapted hunger is so big most of the time that satisfying it just might add some weight. But they don't understand that putting their bodies' fuel needs off constantly by trying to eat so little is actually causing their enlarged appetites, their fears about eating and the loss of control they experience.

The body is designed to take in a substantial number of calories when it runs out of ready fuel. Rice cakes or a handful of carrots do not have substantial calories. Nor do granola bars, bagels, oranges, black coffee or diet drinks. You can medicate your hunger with these things, but you can't satisfy it and get off the Cycle. You'll usually have to eat more, and more substantial food.

Like what?

Cereal with milk. Sandwiches. Pasta dishes. Egg or tofu dishes. Soup with bread. Salads with meat or beans or nuts. Stir-fry and rice. Chili. Look at the Real Foods list or in your favorite broad-spectrum cookbook—it's in there.

Try eating 300 to 600 calories each time you get hungry. That's more substantial than a typical low-cal, no-fat snack. Don't worry about when you last ate—your body knows what it's doing! If you're still hungry after 600, keep eating. You have make-up cravings or extra energy needs to meet, and if you satisfy them now they'll calm down in time, depending on your special body. If you don't satisfy them, they'll never leave you alone.

Of course, if you just want only an orange or a bagel from time to time, then just have that. Always go with your body signals. But most regular healthy eating is in small to medium-sized meal form.

Don't just medicate your hunger, satisfy it.

DIET DOCTRINE #3: Ignoring your hunger is good and necessary and perfectly benign.

Hunger signals are your body's way of telling you it needs fuel. When you ignore your hunger you are telling your body something, too. By not eating, you are telling your body that there is no food available, so it must make do without ready fuel. Your body acquiesces, using muscle tissue and fat for its energy and metabolic needs, but in this process it must also adapt to the famine by gearing up to eventually store fat for future survival. Your appetite increases, your cravings change, your metabolic rate drops, you think more about food and want to move around less.

You thought that ignoring your hunger was beneficial for your weight control. You thought your hunger was your enemy. You believed that it was necessary to go hungry in order to be thin. You thought there was no harm in it.

You were wrong, wrong, wrong, wrong. Ignoring your hunger has brought you to the land of eating trouble. It is not harmless. It is not necessary for natural leanness. It is abusive and leads to pathological eating behaviors and emotional turmoil. Clearly, you need to stop ignoring your hunger.

Perhaps the most destructive consequence of going hungry, besides promoting eating disturbances, is the breakdown of the fuel-need communication system between a person and her body. Hunger is a physical fuel-need distress signal. When it is ignored frequently over time, it becomes distorted in different ways. Undereaters report that they either feel hungry all the time or they never feel hungry anymore. These are examples of two extreme adaptations to the habit of going hungry. It is quite difficult for some people to recover their bodies' natural fuel signals, but they can do it—by learning to listen to their bodies again.

It is physically very stressful to your body to regularly ignore your hunger, and it is a great relief when you stop doing it. Dieters don't realize the impact that going hungry so often has on their energy level, disposition and even sex lives! Ignoring hunger signals is a form of self-abuse that may help keep you artificially thin, but only with the physical and emotional destruction that accompanies the Cycles. How we ever got so far down this anti-hunger road is beyond me.

Hunger satisfaction is the key to your wellness. Never, ever go hungry if you can help it. This is the only way to send your body the message that food is always available and there's consequently no need to store fat. Hunger that is always responded to is hunger that can serve to keep a person lean and healthy. So stop fighting your hunger and take care of it for a change.

Never, ever ignore your hunger again.

DIET DOCTRINE #4: Feeling full should be avoided.

This nonsense goes along with #2, eating as little as possible. Somehow, the natural satisfaction point that people reach when they eat enough eludes the eating disturbed. This has to do with the adaptive breakdown of the natural satisfaction point of chronic undereaters.

When people completely ignore their hunger often, and eat too little the rest of the time, the body has to inspire them to take in big quantities of make-up food when it can. (This happens when undereaters lose control.) In order to accomplish this, their normal satisfaction point becomes blurred. They don't know when they are full. They develop this ability to just eat and eat, even after they are stuffed, and after a while on the Cycle they don't trust their full feelings anymore.

What they don't realize is that they have obliterated their bodies' ability to get full on normal amounts of food. So the term "full" becomes fearful and the feeling is avoided.

When you eat, keep eating high-quality food until you are satisfied, until you feel full. Now, if you've been seriously undereating, you may overeat, not feeling satisfied until you are overfull. That's OK. It'll take awhile. Don't panic if you can help it. Each time you get hungry eat good food until you feel full and want to stop eating. If you overeat you'll know why, and rest assured that it won't last forever.

If you do panic, don't try to do this part yet. Just focus on eating whenever you get hungry. Eating to satisfaction will come later when it won't seem so overwhelming. And, especially for anorectics, eating until you feel full will probably have to come in stages because your body can't take on too much drastic change at once. Just do what you can from day to day and keep the rest of the information for later. It will come back to you when you need it.

Eat Real Food until you are full—then it will be easy to stop.

DIET DOCTRINE #5: Diet foods are best.

When you buy diet foods you get less for your money—fewer calories for more money. It doesn't make sense to me. But what about less fat and less sugar? Aren't these worthy of more money? Only if you're rich and quite lazy.

Diet foods are products of our national obsession with being thin through low-fat, low-sugar and low-calorie food labels. You just don't see all this nonsense in France, England or Italy. Food is food in these countries. And, incidentally, they have lower levels of obesity and eating problems than we do in the United States.

Why have we made these foods so common? Why are they so popular that the food industry can hardly keep up with our demand for them? I'll tell you why. In our country, many of us have become afraid of food. We are afraid of calories, and of fat and of sugar. We think these things make people blow up into physical blobs and we don't want it to happen to us. So we buy foods with reassuring labels that tell us that we won't.

It used to be that carbohydrates caused overweight. Remember *Dr. Atkins' Diet Revolution?* Between-meal snacking was cited as the culprit in weight gain, and mothers chased their little ones out of the kitchen with nothing but a slap on the behind until supper was good and ready. Sugar became the next popular scapegoat to explain why people get fat, not to mention get a host of other problems including depression and poor sex drive!

Just buy regular Real Food!

DIET DOCTRINE #6: Dietary fat is evil.

This latest craze has really taken the low-fat, sugar-free cake: fat makes people fat. It certainly has a logical ring to it, but I don't believe it's true. By itself, dietary fat does not cause people to be fat. Shall I say it again? I said, eating high-fat foods alone doesn't make people fat. Wow.

Now that I've completely shaken one of the most fundamental beliefs in your soul, let me make a few comments about fat in the diet. Dietary fat is helpful to the human body for many reasons. Hunger satisfaction is rarely cited as an important issue for people with weight or eating problems, but I think it is a very significant factor for those trying to get out of food jail. Some dietary fat makes food more tasty. Moreover, meals with some fat are digested more slowly, keeping the body satisfied over a little longer time than meals devoid of fat. With a healthy amount of fat in the diet, people don't have to eat every ninety minutes, but can stay satisfied for three hours or so. Finally, natural fat-soluble vitamins are found in dietary animal and vegetable fat.

When people struggling to overcome eating problems continue to keep fat entirely out of their diets, they usually battle cravings. Fat intake is the last bastion of control, and their bodies send signals that something is missing. We should not just drop everything we've learned about the benefits of lowering dietary fat, but there is a healthful middle ground. Unfortunately, people on the Cycles are not very good at the middle ground. They seem to do better and feel safer at one extreme or another.

So you extremists are probably hoping I'll give you some numerical guidelines for eating fat. Sorry, those numbers are all in your heads. You could probably give a seminar on "Fifty Ways to Leave the Fat Out of Your Diet." You don't need more guidelines to obsess about, you need to change your eating. Now modify your diet to line up with the moderate dietary fat guidelines better.

Some fat is fine. Really.

DIET DOCTRINE #7: Eating between meals is bad.

A rumor got started two or three decades ago that blamed excess weight on between-meal snacks. Somehow, it was thought, those little extras in the midmorning or midafternoon were making people pudgy. I suppose, if you believe that too much eating causes weight gain, you might draw such a conclusion. Of course, it depends on what people are eating at these breaks, but even more on what they're eating, or not eating, at other times.

I have a lot of trouble buying the idea that these snacks, by themselves, ever made people overweight. I'm quite convinced of my position because almost every naturally thin person I have ever interviewed reports eating significant amounts of food between meals every day. And the overweight dieters I coach almost always report that they try not to eat between meals, or if they do, they have only something very light, with few, if any, calories. Go figure.

Intermeal eating is very important for a healthy relationship with food. You're bound to get hungry between mealtimes, so eat then. If you end up not being hungry when the mealtime comes around, don't eat. You're not hungry, right? So wait until you are and then eat again. How does this feel so far?

Mealtime is whenever you're hungry.

DIET DOCTRINE #8: Staying away from food is a helpful weight-control tactic.

Quite a few clients have told me that they keep their refrigerators empty or nearly so. This lack of food definitely affects their at-home eating, although there are some amazing stories of 2 A.M. Twinkie runs to the all-night grocery store and forbidden pizza deliveries at odd hours, too. The major trouble, though, starts when these hungry undereaters leave for the office, or for the movies, or for a party or shopping. (That is, unless the threat becomes too great, and they learn to stay home where it's safe. Anorectics become reclusive this way.) But most undereaters have a way of finding food out there, and their cravings often lead them to rich make-up foods. These dieters usually figure, if they kept food at home too, they'd be eating twice as much. But it's not true, and they suffer from a painful struggle with their runaway appetites, thinking they can't handle having food around in a normal way.

Food avoidance can only go so far in limiting intake in a country where we have food all around. Besides, it's not necessary, and it just pushes the Cycle along, like any undereating trick.

Go to the grocery store today. Buy plenty of good food that you prefer. Don't forget the pasta and potatoes and rice. And juices and eggs and rich whole-grain breads. And stock up on fresh fruits and vegetables, the ones you especially like. And get milk and cereal and soups and crackers. Fill up your refrigerator and cupboards with real, wholesome food, and don't be afraid anymore.

Keep your food stock full.

DIET DOCTRINE #9: You have to exercise to burn off calories so they won't be stored as fat.

Another pervasive modern paranoia about body fat is that any calories that are taken in will be turned into fat unless they are used up in formal, regimented exercise. This belief is linked to other irrational but popular ideas about obesity.

Here it is, late in the twentieth century, and we've decided that our bodies are, unlike animals' bodies, incapable of energy and weight regulation. Even though human bodies have functioned well for thousands of years, our bodies' obvious regulatory mechanisms have been completely ignored by diet propaganda, and people are encouraged to figure out and work off any extra calories they take in, or they believe they are doomed to gain weight.

What a burden. This weight and energy regulation is a full-time job. In fact, it's an impossible full-time job. That's why this internal energy regulator is a standard feature on human bodies. We just aren't designed to do it intellectually, and trying to do it drives us crazy. This is a picture of food jail: trying to do what the body is not designed to do without completely screwing up your eating and appetite.

Exercise. Exercise every day if you like, but please don't try to "burn off" calories so they won't be stored as fat. To do so is simplistic, inaccurate and entrapping. It robs you of the joy of exercise. Exercise to feel better, to improve your stamina, to sleep more soundly. Exercise for fun, for health. Do physical things that you enjoy, but don't worry about burning calories. Your body can handle that so you can have a life.

Energy regulation is your body's job.

HOW TO STOP UNDEREATING: STEP TWO

Having dealt some fatal blows to the basic doctrines of our diet-obsessed culture, we need to fill the void, have some healthy guidelines to replace the destructive ones. The Naturally Thin Program offers a very different set of recommendations, some of which have been mentioned in Step One. Now let's focus on these fundamental teachings to develop our map to freedom from eating problems.

NATURALLY THIN PRESCRIPTION #1: Always eat when you get hungry.

I cannot emphasize enough the potent remedial effect that eating enough good food when you are hungry will have on your eating problem. It seems too simplistic to be so beneficial. Eating enough is the one thing that eating disorders clinics have failed to emphasize with their clients, focusing instead on all sorts of interesting psychological problems. And this is why people are treated over and over again without getting well. These clinics are missing the boat—the food boat.

Learning to eat and never go hungry is the single most important step you can take toward regaining normal, healthy eating. So start doing it, now.

NATURALLY THIN PRESCRIPTION #2: Eat until you feel satisfied.

This is tricky, I know. Some of you never feel satisfied, even after ingesting the entire contents of an industrial-sized refrigerator. So how are you supposed to do this one? Gradually, that's how. The important issue here is to stop undereating, so just keep focused on that. Try eating a meal whenever you get a significant urge for food, and give yourself and your body time to get used to eating again. You may overeat sometimes, you'll surely undereat at times too. Don't panic, this is a learning process, and at least you know why you're overeating now, and that it's self-limiting. You may miss hunger signals altogether at times too. No wonder, you've been ignoring them half your life!

Be patient. Take this a day—no, a meal—at a time. You just can't rush such a big adjustment, even though it's beneficial. Just know that you *can* do it, and keep at it.

NATURALLY THIN PRESCRIPTION #3: Never restrict calories or limit portions.

I can hear you mumbling, "She must be kidding." I'm not. This calorie restriction is the method by which much undereating is accomplished, fueling the Cycles and their negative effects. As long as you're eating quality, nutrient-rich food, you should not worry about amounts. Throw your food scale out now because you're never going to use it again.

Just pile Real Food you like on your plate or in your bowl. Remember, you want to eat high-quality foods to satisfaction, in order to normalize your appetite and eating behavior. Don't worry about ounces or so-called normal servings (they're often tiny). Eat freely. Your body will stop you when you've had enough, and soon you'll stop craving the junk.

NATURALLY THIN PRESCRIPTION #4: Monitor food quality only, eating only high-quality Real Foods.

At last, something you *can* control! This is a touchy area for problem eaters because they tend to abuse this guideline by getting extreme in the way they define high-quality Real Foods. I know many people who believe no-fat, whole-grain cereal and fruit are about the only good foods out there. Once you take away the other control areas, this last legitimate one takes the brunt of leftover control needs.

Most people who have struggled with eating disturbances are at least halfway to degrees as registered dietitians, in terms of their food knowledge. (I know some registered dietitians with eating disorders, too.) This is part of their problem. The more they know about food, the more anxiety and control problems they have, the worse their eating problems grow. The only information they can really use to help them get well is their knowledge of a balanced diet, period. This gives them some idea of what they are shooting for, but the negative side of this knowledge is usually dominant. These nutritionist types have a hard time shaking all the daily requirements and international units out of their heads. They need to ignore much of their "knowledge" and use only the basics of what they know to choose good food. (Real Foods are listed in the Appendix, pages 277–280.

NATURALLY THIN PRESCRIPTION #5: Keep quality food with you at all times.

After dieting nothing contributes to undereating more than poor food availability. You're hungry, and there's nothing to eat, or there's nothing decent to eat. So you don't eat, or you eat lousy foods. What can you do?

Take it with you. Take food to your office. Take it in your car. Pack a lunch or two and take it to work, or to the mall or to the seminar. Don't let yourself get hungry and stranded without good food. Hunger forces your body into that adaptation mode you're trying to stop. If you want your body to adjust to a new no-famine routine, then you must eliminate the famines by having good food around to eat whenever and wherever you get hungry. You *can* take it with you. Do.

NATURALLY THIN PRESCRIPTION #6: Eat a broad-based diet with emphasis on whole grains, fruits, vegetables and lean protein foods.

"Broad-based" means "spanning all food groups," including grains and cereals, fruits and vegetables, meat and poultry and dairy products. Of course, if you have food allergies or sensitivities, or you are vegetarian, you can easily make those adjustments.

This is a very general recommendation, meant to help you relax your eating controls.

One of the common methods by which undereaters keep their eating under control is to eliminate whole food groups from their diets. Many vegetarians I have interviewed gave up meat in order to lose weight. And dieters everywhere have eliminated or restricted bread, potatoes or pasta to tackle their weight problems. Now it's popular to eliminate fats, which is not really a food group at all. But in order to do it, meats and dairy products must be seriously curtailed.

Eating should be pleasant and, unless you have medical restrictions, free from inordinate rules and regulations. You should be free to eat a meal almost anywhere you go, and free to prepare meals with a wide variety of delicious foods. You shouldn't have to worry much about grams of this or grams of that, completed proteins or partial carbohydrates. A plate of good food should look appetizing, not like a bunch of food-value equations. Don't laugh, you know this is a problem for some of you.

Try letting go of your policeman's role in your eating. Relax. It's OK to like to eat and it's OK to eat foods you enjoy. Eat a variety of Real Foods that you like.

NATURALLY THIN PRESCRIPTION #7: Keep a moderate exercise schedule.

Exercise would be considered moderate if it averages anywhere between thirty minutes three times a week to one hour daily six days a week. This includes sports, weight training, aerobics, walking and fitness machines. If you're exercising moderately now, great. If your exercise is excessive (much more than an hour daily), then moderate gradually if you feel it's out of balance. You can cut back fifteen minutes every week or so until you're within a moderate range. If you're addicted to exercise, you may need some help and support in order to do this. To find out if you're addicted, try cutting back. If you have withdrawal symptoms (anxiety, preoccupation or increased fear of eating) or you can't cut back, see a therapist and stop using that computerized calorimeter.

If you aren't exercising at all, get started. It's important for your recovery, not because it helps control weight, but because it helps manage fear. Exercise uses up some of that excessive energy that accompanies anxiety, and you're bound to be having some anxiety as you make progress toward normal eating. Plus, most people who are more physically active feel less afraid of eating when they get hungry.

Try to resist the temptation to exercise in response to your fear of weight gain, as a way of purging food you have eaten. This will only keep the Cycle kindled. Your goal here is to develop a healthy relationship with your physical activity level, along with sensible eating. It's a lot to balance, but you can do it.

NATURALLY THIN PRESCRIPTION #8: Throw your scale away.

Knowing your weight from day to day will only fuel your fear of food and keep you locked into the Cycle you're on. Don't allow its influence on your eating behavior anymore. There are just too many other important things to think about besides the stupid little numbers on that magnifying dial. It may seem like a trivial thing, but the status of the scale can make or break recovery for some. Don't minimize its influence on your life. Toss your scale out—you'll be glad you did.

Where Do You Stand Now?

Check any statements that describe where the information here has led you so far. Be honest; this is for you.

__ I completely agree with just about everything I've read and I'm ready to apply these principles to my eating.

__ Most of this makes sense to me and I think I'll try some suggestions although, I admit, I'm scared.

__ I know these things are probably true, but I'm just not ready to change. I can't let go right now, but I want to keep learning because I know that, sooner or later, I'll have to face them.

__ I agree with most of the book so far, but I still think my eating problems are psychological, too, so I'm unsure about trying these suggestions.

__ I understand what the book is saying, but there's no way I'm going to risk gaining weight just to have normal eating.

__ The information here is such a relief because I finally have hope for overcoming my eating problem.

__ I have already started applying these principles to my eating because I know they are true.

__ I spent time and money in therapy for my eating disorder, and I am getting angry because they never told me these things about my body.

If I missed where you're at, write it down here. It's important to know where we are if we're planning to make progress from there.

Don't judge yourself based on the information you're learning here. You can get well from the unlikeliest place, believe me. Many have done it.

SUPPORT NEEDS

One of the disadvantages of the Naturally Thin Program at this time is its lack of a support network. There are plenty of eating disorders groups, clinics and even hospitals that are psychologically oriented. But they can't help you because you're not dealing with emotional issues; you're learning to eat. And there's not much out there to help people learn to eat, so where do you go for support?

You go to your own life resources. You acknowledge your need for support and then you creatively find places to get it within your familial, social, spiritual and personal resources. First, you have to identify these resources, and then you have to solicit and develop the support you need.

Identifying Resources of Support

People you ask to support you in your quest for normal eating should read this book or, at the very least, understand its premise and your goals. After that, the main task of a Naturally Thin support person is reassurance—reassurance that you are still OK even though you are eating, reassurance that you still look fine when you feel like a blob, reassurance that you are not going to gain a hundred pounds in two weeks and reassurance that these principles are rational steps to breaking out of food jail.

Most clients know where they can get support, and where they can't, in their families. Some have no one in their families they can count on. Others are confident of one or two family members. But they are rare. This just seems to be a problem a bit too close to home for most.

Friends seem to be better able and willing to support their friends in this eating adventure. Some are definitely better at this than others, so choose friends whom you respect and who respect you—those with whom you don't have inordinate control or enmeshment struggles.

Spiritual sources of support abound and come in many different styles, though we may forget their importance as practical advisers in our daily lives. Your faith can play a tremendous role in your recovery. Because one of the main challenges of the Naturally Thin Program is anxiety, prayer or meditation and the application of spiritual principles can attenuate this fear, helping you to maintain hope and persevere.

Your own intelligence and problem-solving abilities are resources, too. When you are struggling and need a boost, you can consider what you can do to help yourself. Perhaps rereading this book, or sections of it, will give you a lift. Or make a chart of your progress for encouragement. You can review the successes and symptoms of improvement that you've experienced for self-support. The list is long if you want to help yourself.

AN EXERCISE FOR THE READER

Take two pieces of paper. On one write down the nine diet doctrines in this chapter. Read them out loud, one at a time, and then cross them out, one by one. Burn the paper or tear it up and put it in the garbage.

Now take the other paper and write out the eight Naturally Thin Prescriptions. Read them out loud, one at a time, and then underline them, one by one. Fold the paper and put it in your purse or billfold. Take it out and read it when you need it.

CHAPTER 5

Getting Out of Jail

TRADITIONAL DIET TACTICS ARE BASED ON THE IDEA that weight must be managed through permanent, intellectually controlled food restriction because bodies can't be trusted with unlimited food. According to diet experts, bingeing behavior, cravings for sweets and fatty foods, and food preoccupation are simply hard-core evidence of the body's incompetence in regulating food intake to maintain healthy weight.

The mind-controlled famine diet is like a jail sentence of life without parole. Although promising thinness and relief from weight problems, dieting is itself directly responsible for causing the adaptive adjustments in hunger and appetite that lock victims into eating disturbances. Isn't it ironic? Rather than symptoms of incompetence, these adjustments are actually brilliant displays of the body's sensitive adaptability to diversities in the food supply.

NATURALLY THIN PROGRAM VS. TRADITIONAL DIETING

The main difference between traditional dieting and the Naturally Thin Program is the *focus of control* for eating. Traditional dieting presumes that the mind must control eating behavior because the body cannot be trusted to eat the right amount of food at the right time. In contrast, Naturally Thin is a *body-controlled* eating program because, as traditional dieting has illustrated so clearly, the mind is not designed to control eating behavior. Eating is visceral and under the body's domain. When we try to force our bodies to eat according to when and how much we think we should, based on a mind-designed diet, we get caught in the Feast or Famine Cycle, and end up feeling crazy, eating out of control and miserable.

ELIMINATING FAMINES

The Naturally Thin Program targets this problem of eliminating famines by teaching people how to eat enough good food when they need it. There are two kinds of famines to eliminate: *quantity famines,* which we are all familiar with (undereating); and *quality famines,* which are about poor-quality food. People in quality famines may eat when they are hungry, but they eat food with poor nutrient value.

The standard for eating enough at the right time must be based not on objective intellectual values, but on the subjective signals of individual bodies. Food quality, on the other hand, is determined intellectually. But appetite and variations in food interest must play a role in choosing from among quality foods in order for the body to be satisfied.

In this chapter, you're going to learn how to turn control for your eating back over to your body, and how to abandon the intellectual control you have exerted over your appetite and eating (except for controlling food quality). The decisions of when and how much food to eat are transferred to the jurisdiction of the body, and must be governed by fuel-need (hunger) and fuel-full (satisfaction) signals alone. This is the only way to eliminate the famine experience that leads to eating disturbances. When the famines are eliminated the body can readapt to the new food supply by normalizing the appetite, metabolism and weight.

HOW TO TURN EATING CONTROLS OVER TO YOUR BODY

Again, undoing the diet lifestyle that keeps your eating crazy boils down to one basic shift: moving the center for eating control from your mind to your body. This shift from mind to body control must be fairly complete if you want to enjoy a normal relationship with food. The rest of the diet lifestyle usually fades with time away from overcontrolled eating habits.

How, exactly, do you undo the mental control you have learned to exert on your eating behavior? And then, how do you learn to allow your body signals to govern your eating?

MAKING THE EATING CONTROL SHIFT

The Naturally Thin Program opposes the foundation of traditional dieting. Unlike the traditional dieter who ignores hunger and tries to eat less than the appetite calls for, the person breaking out of food jail must learn to stop ignoring hunger signals and tune into them, eating to satisfaction every time hunger strikes. Hunger signals that have long gone unsatisfied or undersatisfied are sometimes relentless during the first weeks, but as they are consistently satisfied, they usually moderate within a few days to several weeks.

Bear in mind, if you are anorectic or extremely frightened of giving up any control over your eating, you will do better if you integrate these recommendations gradually and with support. Contact a professional for help.

STARTING THE CONTROL SHIFT

Getting started is often the trickiest part of learning body-controlled eating. Iris, a client who was anxious to get it right from the beginning, asked me for specific instructions. Here's our conversation:

JEAN: Get up in the morning and go to the kitchen. Always go directly to the fuel room first thing. Ask yourself, Am I hungry?

If the answer is no, look at some appetizing food. If it looks good to you, that's enough of a quiet hunger signal. Eat. But if it still isn't appealing, just go back and look at good food about every hour until you *do* want to eat. (I call this "presenting food.") Some bodies have to be coaxed a little.

When the answer is, Yes, I'm hungry, what next? don't try to figure out whether or not you *should* be hungry or whether your hunger merits eating. It doesn't matter how hungry you are because any degree of hunger is a signal that deserves a response.

IRIS: I think, I should have a piece of fruit because it's fat-free and one diet expert whom I know of says fruit is the only type of food your body can digest in the morning.

JEAN: Wait! You're thinking too much. Do you *want* fruit? Does fruit sound good *to your body?*

IRIS: Well, no, not really. I *want* a bowl of cereal, and I *want* toast and orange juice.

JEAN: Now you're talking. Eat that—as much as you want. Don't stop eating until you really feel full and want to stop.

IRIS: But what if I *want* fruit?

JEAN: Then have it, of course. As much as you like, and cereal and toast too, if you want that.

IRIS: What if I don't think about eating because I'm not that hungry?

JEAN: Then you must stop and listen to your body more carefully. Even a little hunger is a signal that you need fuel—as long as food is appealing. If you're a little hungry but nothing looks good, wait awhile. Have something light when your hunger is light.

IRIS: Like what?

JEAN: Like a muffin or bagel and juice. Try to discover what you're hungry for. What sounds good?

IRIS: And what if I'm hungry for a huge, greasy caramel roll, or ten?

JEAN: Here's where the thinking comes in. You know that caramel rolls are poor-quality food. So think about what else—something like a caramel roll but of higher quality—sounds good, like toasted raisin-nut bread with butter and cinnamon-sugar. Then have that. Any foods on the Real Foods list are OK and, if you're going to eat rich food, do it in the morning.

IRIS: What about limits? How do I decide *how much* I should eat?

JEAN: That depends on how hungry you are. In general, the hungrier you are, the more you are likely to eat—but not always. You eat until you *want* to stop eating, *and not before.* You eat until you look at the food and you know you don't want anymore. You don't stuff yourself, but you don't stop until you really *want* to stop eating.

This doesn't mean that you stop when you start getting afraid of how much you are eating (unless you need to take these steps very gradually—then go as far as you can). And it doesn't mean you stop eating when you *think* you've eaten enough. And it doesn't mean that you stop eating when you've eaten what you consider a normal amount of food. You stop only *when your body tells you to stop* by means of its fuel-full signals. It's easy to stop when your body stops you.

IRIS: What if I have a whole bowl of cereal and toast and juice and I'm still hungry? I can't just keep eating, can I?

JEAN: Yes, you can. But it may trigger too much fear at first. Eventually, you must, if you want to be free from your eating problems. If you can, keep eating until your body stops you. Your body *will* stop you when it is satisfied.

This is your goal: to completely satisfy your body's need for fuel whenever it signals a need all day long every day.

IRIS: OK. What next? What do I have for lunch?

JEAN: Wait a minute, it's only 7:15 A.M. at breakfast time, and you'll be hungry again before lunch, which is at least four hours away, especially if you're working in an office environment. You'll need to eat before lunch—call it a "second feeding."

IRIS: When?

JEAN: When your body asks for it.

IRIS: When is that? I've got to be able to plan a little, you know.

JEAN: Usually bodies that are fed high-quality low-fat meals on demand need food about every two or three hours. This depends on activity level, calories eaten at a sitting, size of the person, basal metabolic rate and probably a dozen other factors that we know little about. Many naturally thin people eat four to six meals a day.

IRIS: Oh, I get it, this is the six-small-meals-a-day diet.

JEAN: No, it's not. If you control your intake (have small meals) or the number of times you eat (six) because of fear, you won't get well. Remember, your goal is to let your body control when and how much you eat. You've been demoted to one simple job: to restrict your food choices to quality food only. Let's say you get hungry again at 9:45 A.M. Time for the second feeding.

IRIS: Nine forty-five! I just ate. It's been only two hours since I ate breakfast.

JEAN: The time doesn't matter. And it doesn't matter how long it's been since you last ate. You are hungry and that's all that matters. You will eat.

IRIS: I'm at work then. There's nothing to eat there.

JEAN: Then you'll have to take your second feeding with you. You know, pack a brunch.

IRIS: I get it. But I'll have to keep food with me for my feedings throughout the rest of the day, too, so I don't miss any hunger signals and end up in a famine, right?

JEAN: Very good! Your second feeding, just like the first, should be high-quality food you want, and as much as you want to eat. You'll be hungry again in a few hours anyway. Do the same thing again at lunchtime, and again in the middle or late afternoon. By dinnertime, you should have eaten at least three meals already and you shouldn't be ravenous if you've stayed "fed up"—kept up with your body's demands for fuel.

The first weeks you may still feel quite hungry at dinner. Some-times, when a newly liberated body gets the message that there's finally enough food available, the hunger signals really intensify for a while. Try not to panic. They *will* settle down as you keep eating well.

IRIS: What if there are donuts or cake in the office at my break times?

JEAN: Never eat poor-quality food unless you don't have any choice. This is why taking food with you for all day eating is so im-portant—so you don't get stranded without a choice. After dinner (your fourth, fifth or sixth meal—preferably eaten in the early evening), you can handle a little hunger if you're not active at this time. Here is your one chance to be in control. Mild hunger (toler-able, doesn't interfere with your sleep) before bedtime should be manageable with light snacks like fruit, toast and cereal, if you feel you need to eat. This is no time for pizza! (Breakfast is the best time for pizza!)

THE NATURALLY THIN PROGRAM:
BODY-CONTROLLED EATING

This is a condensation of the Naturally Thin Program for break-ing out of food jail. By now, it may feel like a review, but it is very important to go over the main points again.

- Tune into your hunger signals.
- Always eat nutrient-packed food whenever you get hungry until you are completely satisfied.
- Never, ever let your body get overly hungry.
- Choose foods you want to eat from the high-quality Real Foods list.
- Keep high-quality foods with you so you won't get famished.
- Don't worry about the clock—eat when you are hungry.
- Do not limit portions.
- Never ignore hunger, except after dinner if it's mild and you are inactive.
- Don't restrict your eating by limiting groups of foods, unless you are allergic. Eat a variety of foods.

One More Time, Just to Be Sure

Eat as much high-quality Real Food as you need to satisfy your body's hunger all day long every day. *Never go hungry,* but eat only quality calories, according to your body's hunger signals. Take cues for when to eat, and how much to eat, only from your body. Decide what to eat based on what you're hungry for, plus the foods you know are high quality.

When you make these eating changes, you "move" from a famine environment to an environment of "optimal food availability," and you may overeat for a while. You may experience an excessive appetite and gain some weight. This is because your body is still programmed by your past undereating to store up for the famines of the future, and your letting go of the controls is its cue to begin stocking your fat reserves. If you have recently lost quite a lot of weight by dieting, you may want to consult your doctor to monitor your readaptation. If you have any medical problems even remotely related to your diet, check with your doctor before starting. Take this book to your appointment and ask your doctor to supervise you.

EATING ON TIME

Eating well is about quality calories, but "eating on time" is about staying tuned in to your body's fuel needs; it has nothing to do with the time. Eating on time is the opposite of "eating late." When you eat on time you eat as soon as you get hungry. For those of you who are purists, that means, ideally, eating within five minutes of a hunger signal if you are physically active, and within fifteen minutes if you are at rest. Eating on time is the cornerstone of getting off the Cycles because the quick response to hunger is the only means of consistently eliminating famines. Eating late, on the other hand, is something Cyclers are used to—ignoring hunger and eating long after hunger signals are perceived. Even a half hour is a long time for your body to wait for food when it is out of fuel.

Three Basic Skills of Body-Controlled Eating

1. *when* to eat: **whenever you are hungry,** probably *more often* than you are used to

2. how *much* to eat: **enough to satisfy your hunger**—*more* food than you are used to eating regularly, especially early in the day

3. *what* to eat: **exclusively high-quality Real Food**—perhaps *better food* than you've been eating, and/or *more variety with fewer restrictions* (when you're eating enough it is not difficult to limit yourself to quality food only)

Numbers 1 and 2, when and how much you eat, are to be controlled completely by your body because it is designed to regulate food intake. Did you know that there is no known obesity in animals in the wild? And it's not because food is always naturally limited—it often isn't. It's because animals eat instinctively. Fortunately, they can't interfere with their natural eating urges the way we can.

Number 3, what you eat, has to be a cooperative effort between you and your body. Your body will lead you to different foods via its appetite changes, cravings and aversions. You follow your body's lead, but keep quality, variety and balance in mind, too, when deciding what to eat. For example, you've already had two sandwiches one day, and although another sounds appealing, you decide on something different that sounds good as well, like a chicken Caesar salad and fruit, or pasta with vegetables. You're not ignoring your body's signals, you're simply using your head to enhance your diet.

EATING PATTERNS DURING THE SHIFT TO BODY CONTROL

Former undereaters who have gotten off the Cycles tend to eat in similar patterns. They are usually hungry every two or three hours, they tend to eat a meal of sorts each time they get hungry, and they eat between four and seven meals a day.

During the first days or weeks of the Naturally Thin Program, ex-undereaters may crave foods that have been restricted while they were cycling. The most common Real Food cravings are for breads, juices, cereals, eggs, meats, butter and mayonnaise. The high-fat foods may be desired because of the lingering need for fat, but the complex carbohydrate cravings are also certainly related to the senseless overlimiting of these healthful foods during periods of restricted eating.

Of course, former undereaters also might continue to want old make-up favorites like ice cream, frozen yogurt, chips, pastries and candies. These cravings are also related to undereating and should be completely gone within a few weeks of quality on-time eating, unless there has been a significant weight loss from dieting, or anorexia and underweight. Then the cravings may continue for a longer time. Of course, these cravings will never cease unless you get off the Cycle! (More on this in the Recovery Timetable, page 134.)

What should you do about these cravings? Should you indulge yourself? Does your body really need these foods?

EARLY CRAVINGS FOR SWEETS AND FATS

It seems that common sense should answer these questions, but I've been asked so many times that I am convinced that many ex-faminers really do need advice here. It's easier to prevent weight gain than to reverse it. If you're interested in minimizing the initial weight gain that some ex-faminers experience in getting off their Cycles (and you can only get off the Cycles from the feasting phase), then don't indulge your body's cravings for poor-quality sweet and fatty foods. You may overeat somewhat in the first few weeks, but you and your body will be much further along in recovery if you allow yourself only Real Foods to feast on.

There are plenty of richer foods on the Real Foods list from which to choose that will help satisfy these cravings, and by choosing them you'll be practicing an important essential of healthful eating from day one: controlling the food availability factor (FAF). The Naturally Thin Program allows you to keep only high-quality Real Food around because Borderline and Pleasure Foods (listed in the Appendix, pages 277–280) do not meet your body's fuel needs adequately to force normalization of appetite and eating. These poor-quality foods cause quality famines, and famines of any kind—quantity or quality—keep the Cycles and all their symptoms going. So eat well from the very beginning and you'll break the Cycle you are on as quickly as possible.

GETTING OFF THE CYCLE: WHAT ABOUT FAT?

A high-quality diet is lower in fat. This is why I suggest that you avoid high-fat foods from the start. Of course, if you are eating no-fat or extremely low-fat, you need to add some fat to get your diet in balance to break the Cycle. A lower-fat (not no-fat!) eating program gives your body the strongest signal that the food supply is optimal. Remember, high-fat eating causes quality famines because fatty foods aren't as nutrient-rich as leaner foods, but they are important for balance and diet satisfaction. I've found that clients who swear off Borderline Foods, avoid fattier foods on the Real Foods list, and bulk up with abandon on whole grains, fruits, vegetables, lean meats and lower fat dairy products get off the Feast or Famine Cycle fastest and stay off.

Sometimes former faminers have a decided distaste for vegetables, salads and other no-fat snacks at the beginning of their new eating program. This makes sense in light of the fact that they have often forced themselves to eat these "perfect" diet foods ad nauseam. They are overloaded! This aversion concerns some people because they know that vegetables are nutrient-rich and that they should eat them. Don't worry if you find yourself hating leafy greens at this stage. Your cravings for these wonderful foods will develop as your body adjusts to having enough good food for a change.

Often people getting off the Cycles crave bread for a few weeks, some as much as a loaf a day! Other bread products that have been on the forbidden list a long time also become favorites at this stage: English muffins, bagels, bread sticks, etc. Should you indulge these cravings? Yes! Bread products, especially from whole grains, can be excellent sources of fiber and nutrients. But try to fit in plenty of other sources of complex carbohydrates, too—pasta, rice and potatoes.

EATING ENOUGH: CHANGING YOUR BODY'S ADAPTIVE RESPONSES

Remember the five adaptive responses to undereating described in Chapter 2? They are a lowered metabolic rate, the urge to overeat, cravings for sweets and/or fatty foods, preoccupation with food and eating, and depressed physical energy. These adaptive responses parallel most symptoms of disturbed eating. Even body-image distortion seems to be an adaptive response of sorts (more on this in Chapter 6). If you have experienced any or all of these five adaptive responses, regardless of your other symptoms, your body has been struggling to keep you alive in spite of your undereating.

Let's go back to the cause of these five adaptive responses: inadequate food intake. Low food intake is the environmental stimulus that provokes these unique adaptations, just as sunlight exposure provokes the adaptive pigmentation of skin. If you want to change the way your body is adapting, you have to start by understanding what environmental stimulus provokes the adaptive responses. And in order to eliminate adaptive responses, you must change the stimulus that provokes them.

For example, a person who wants to stop the adaptive tanning response would logically avoid exposure to sunlight. This seems obvious to everyone who knows that changes in pigmentation of the skin are stimulated by exposure to sunlight. But consider what someone who is unaware of this fact might do. She might try bathing more often, using a moisturizer to wash off the tan or even going to a psychotherapist. You can't really blame her; she just doesn't know.

> **No matter what you do to get over your eating problem, if you keep undereating you will stay trapped.**

And if you are determined to continue to undereat, you'll probably have to use a lot of energy just to keep coping with your body's adaptive mechanisms. At least now you'll understand the endless conflict, bizarre eating patterns and powerful control struggles you experience.

REVERSING THE ADAPTIVE TREND

To change the ways your body is adapting to its food supply, you must change this supply. If you keep trying to limit your eating, you will find yourself locked in a physical war with your body because of its innate adaptive responses.

We've discussed why you should stop going hungry and how to

go about doing that. Making these eating changes will lead you out of food jail and into normal eating. Now let's take a look at exactly how this happens. What goes on inside your body when you give it enough food day in and day out, week after week and month after month?

If you "move" to an environment where good food is always available, by always eating quality food in response to your hunger, the five adaptive responses to undereating you have experienced will gradually *reverse*. These adaptations are all basic symptoms of eating disturbances. The only way to get out of food jail is to systematically eat enough. The only way.

If you're underweight, you'll gain some weight. You need to. But you can now have confidence that you'll not gain indefinitely, and will eventually level off at a healthy weight for your height, bone structure and activity level. And if you're overweight, your body will very gradually work to eliminate excess fat. If your weight is just about right, you may gain at first, too, and then return to your ideal weight, free of your eating struggles. Here's how it works.

READAPTATION

When you "leave" a famine environment, your body again experiences biochemical changes because the fuel supply is now continuous. Remember, gearing up to store fat is not adaptive (supporting survival) for bodies that get plenty of good food on time. So your body is faced with the physiological challenge of readaptation—to reverse the five adaptive responses it developed during the famine times.

These are the body's five adaptive responses to a continuous supply of high-quality food:

1. elevated metabolic rate
2. normalization of appetite, intolerance of bingeing and overeating
3. cravings for nutrient-rich foods and intolerance for sweets and fatty foods
4. disinterest in food and eating (diet boredom)
5. increased desire for physical activity

These are biochemically controlled responses to the continuous availability of quality food. Your body can be reprogrammed to stop its fat production efforts. The key is a continuous high-quality food supply over time. (Changes in adaptation are gradual and body weight adjustments usually take several years to be completed.)

RESULTS OF PERSISTENT BODY-CONTROLLED EATING

Let's take a look at each of these adaptive responses to a continuous supply of good-quality food:

1. Elevated Metabolic Rate:

Most people, and certainly those with eating disturbances, know that there's one surefire way to stimulate the metabolism (get the body to burn calories faster): exercise. But few people, I have found, know a different and very effective way to rev up the body's engine: eating. Eating? Yes, eating stimulates the body's metabolic rate, causing it to burn calories at a faster rate. It's the same principle at work as stoking a fire: add fuel and you automatically increase combustion. The body receiving regular doses of fuel does not have to conserve—it can hum along at an optimal metabolic speed, even wasting calories in heat. It doesn't have to be as energy efficient as the underfed body. Besides this effect, the digestive process itself is fueled by calories from food, so some calories consumed are "wasted" in making food useful to the body. So there are really two main methods for stimulating the metabolic rate: exercise and eating. Don't sabotage your exercise benefits by shortchanging your body's fuel supply!

2. Normalization of Appetite, Intolerance of Bingeing and Overeating:

Just as undereaters tend to develop exaggerated appetites as adaptative responses to the lack of food, people who eat enough on a regular basis do not, in fact, cannot overeat. The enlarged appetite of an undereater can only decrease to a normal level if the food intake becomes truly adequate and is maintained over time. Those who suffer from disturbed eating have a hard time believing it will, but the proof of this principle is demonstrated in their own bodies. After eating enough for a while, they themselves experience this normalization of appetite, and I don't have to try to convince them anymore. This often heralds the beginning of a new confidence in their bodies.

This principle is so evident in naturally thin people, who are commonly reputed to eat a lot of food and often. It is not unusual for them to feel embarrassed by their apparent immunity from weight problems. Not infrequently they are victims of envy and anger because dieters think that natural thins are simply blessed with magical metabolisms that keep them thin in spite of their bountiful eating behavior. What they don't realize is this: Abundant, instinctive, generous eating keeps these people so svelte. They couldn't binge if they wanted to. They are too full from eating so well so often all day long every day. Bingeing and overeating, I have observed, are only practiced and well tolerated by people who go hungry.

3. Cravings for Nutrient-Rich Foods, and Intolerance for Sweets and Fatty Foods:

When a starving body gets plenty of good food, its needs and priorities change. Fat becomes unnecessary and maladaptive. Excess fat on well-fed bodies is burdensome, working against survival, so cravings shift to high-quality foods packed with nutrients to optimize. Ex-undereaters develop a decided intolerance for, even an aversion to, the old fat producers they craved when they were starving. These foods don't satisfy the body's new need for adaptive leanness and health. Metabolism-stimulating, nutrient-rich, high-quality foods do.

4. Disinterest in Food and Eating (Diet Boredom):

Eating behavior becomes the central focal point of living for people who are undereating or starving. This adaptation is clearly linked to eating avoidance because it is simply not experienced by people who eat enough as a routine, something that eating-disturbed individuals and dieters can hardly imagine. Even normal-weight volunteers without eating problems who are underfed report a total preoccupation with food.

Diet boredom is a surprising relief for people recovering from eating struggles since they are usually weary of having their lives revolve around food, eating and weight-control issues. They are especially glad to see their attention turning toward other, more important concerns, and relieved that their diet focus is not some mysterious evidence of an obsessive psychological disorder. The fact that it disappears by simply increasing regular food intake is proof of its adaptive and physical nature.

5. Increased Desire for Physical Activity:

When a body that has adapted to inadequate food finally gets enough food on a regular basis, the baseline energy level naturally goes up. The new food supply, once it is established as a long-term change, allows for energy waste rather than strict conservation. One of the major manifestations of this shift is in the area of movement motivation. Generally, people who eat plenty of good food all day experience a greater inclination to be physically active than people who undereat or eat poor-quality food erratically.

The human body is designed with motion in mind, and medical scientists have been touting the multiple benefits of regular exercise, especially in the last decade. There is no doubt that moving around more is good for everyone—that is, unless you haven't got enough fuel to supply the movement. Most people agree that they should exercise more, but relatively few ever get around to it regularly. I think this has more to do with our terrible eating habits (and eating-avoidance habits) than our characters.

Well-fed bodies like to move around. It feels natural and good. It is energizing rather than draining, as well as health-promoting. People whose food supply is adequate report *cravings* for exercise just as underfed exercisers complain of relentless cravings for calorie-rich food. Bodies know what they need and are persistently trying to tell us.

WHEN BODIES ARE IN CONTROL OF EATING

In contrast to the three Cycles we've discussed, body-controlled eating puts a person on a path straight out of the food trap. Here's an illustration of that path, including the changes that occur as a result of this control shift.

SHIFT FROM INTELLECTUAL TO BODY-CONTROLLED EATING

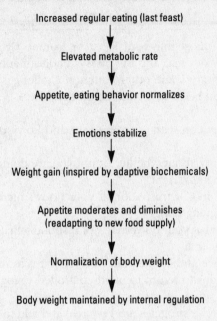

Increased regular eating (last feast)

↓

Elevated metabolic rate

↓

Appetite, eating behavior normalizes

↓

Emotions stabilize

↓

Weight gain (inspired by adaptive biochemicals)

↓

Appetite moderates and diminishes
(readapting to new food supply)

↓

Normalization of body weight

↓

Body weight maintained by internal regulation

There is no Cycle, no rebound effect or loss of control on this path.

By giving the eating controls back to your body, you force it to readapt to a new environmental stress: optimal food supply. You'll be surprised at how quickly your body can begin to respond to having the controls.

"But," you protest, "I can't let *my* body control my eating—I'd be a blimp in no time! You don't know my appetite. It's absolutely insatiable! How can you expect me to let go of these controls? I'm terrified of letting go. Isn't that why people with eating disturbances have such crazy eating habits in the first place?"

Yes, it is. These are very good questions and the answers are not as complicated as you might think. Hang on, this is scary, I know, but this is the path out of food jail. It may help you to know that everyone who takes the Naturally Thin path to freedom from eating problems is frightened. Some are absolutely terrified. And guess what? Many do it anyway, because they are so very tired of living in the hellhole of pathological eating, and there is simply no other way out.

WITHDRAWAL SYMPTOMS GETTING OFF THE CYCLES

Fear is the most universal Feast or Famine Cycle withdrawal symptom. Besides fear and the physical adjustments your body is making, there are some other common challenges that you may develop as you become a body-controlled eater:

1. preoccupation with your recovery and how your body is responding
2. uncertainty about whether or not you are doing the Naturally Thin Program "right"
3. surprise and/or frustration at your body's increasing intolerance of going hungry
4. concern that your body may not respond—that it really is defective after all
5. impatience at the time your body requires to readapt
6. temptations to return to mind-controlled eating

Although these struggles are very real and add to the distress of making the shift to body-controlled eating, it is fear that challenges people with disturbed eating the most. And fear is really the feature that lies behind all six withdrawal symptoms. So what can you do about the fear?

DEPROGRAMMING FEAR

The most potent antidotes to fear are knowledge, faith and support. But in order to be effective, the knowledge must be true, the faith based on truth and the source of support aware of the truth. These three are effective for combating fear, especially paralyzing fear that prevents people from following what they want to do and know is right. When you are paralyzed with fear, you are unable to act in spite of your desire. You know you need to keep your body satisfied, but you are so frightened of gaining weight that you just can't.

Knowledge is very important in coping with fear because much fear is based on ignorance or partial knowledge, and thorough knowledge or information is usually reassuring. It has a calming effect. Knowledge itself can increase security. So when fear comes a-knockin' at your door—fear of food, fear of fat, fear of letting go, of losing control—get back into this book and remind yourself of what you're doing and why, and how much sense it really makes.

Powerful faith can be activated to make a bridge over your fear, between your goal and the things you need to do to reach it. "Faith is the evidence of things hoped for, the confidence in things yet unseen," writes Saint Paul. You can learn to rely on your faith to develop a normal eating lifestyle as a source of hope and confidence in your recovery. But this faith must be nurtured and exercised to make it strong. How? By using it as a source of strength. Oddly, like your muscles, faith is increased best by using it most. When you are afraid, seek ways to tap your faith—pray for inner peace, meditate on the liberty you seek, contemplate the path you are taking to wholeness—whatever method works for you to cope with your fear. Let your faith fill your mind and heart with confidence.

There's nothing quite like a reassuring face and voice to calm fears and help you regain your emotional bearings. A supportive friend who is familiar with the Naturally Thin Program can turn a panic attack into a resistible temptation, often in a simple conversation. Use your support system when you feel your emotions slipping out from under you.

WITHDRAWAL SYMPTOMS

Barbara could hardly believe she had agreed to try the Naturally Thin Program—she was still convinced that her bingeing and purging were psychological. She knew they would continue as long as her anger did, no matter what she ate. But she agreed to try it anyway. She said she wanted me to be wrong so she wouldn't feel so bad about the $16,000 she had spent in therapy for her bulimia over the years.

Although she felt terrified of letting go and eating more, Barbara took the plunge with courage. One trick she used that helped her was this: Whenever she got scared, she would say to herself, This is voluntary. I can go back to controlling my eating anytime. I've been doing that for almost ten years, and look where I am. This is worth a serious try, if only to prove that it is emotional, so I'm not going to let this fear thing

stop me. This self-talk was usually just the boost Barbara
needed to keep going. I called it her "heartening speech."

Barbara didn't have an easy road breaking out of food
jail, but her bingeing and purging stopped completely during
her fourth week. Once completely off the Cycle, Barbara had
other challenges and fears to deal with, but she never, ever
went back to the binge/purge nightmare that took her out of
life for nearly a decade.

EVERYONE ENDS THE CYCLE WITH A FEAST

People with eating disturbances are fearful and sometimes phobic about weight gain, so the idea of gaining at first can be a real
problem. Let's understand why ex-undereaters sometimes gain
weight temporarily.

Those brave souls who begin to allow their bodies to control
their eating voluntarily on this program usually have make-up eating to do. They have biochemicals in their bodies that promote fat
storage because of their undereating and consequent adaptive responses. These biochemicals do not automatically go away because of a decision to stop famining. The body doesn't "know" the
famines are over forever. It has been programmed to prepare for
famines, and that's what it will do once the last undereating ends
and food "becomes available." So when the undereater starts to eat
enough, often the adaptive overeating starts, too, and the urge to
overeat and cravings for fat-producing foods remain for a time.

This is why ex-faminers gain weight or plateau for a while before they level off at their ideal weight. Your body doesn't trust the
environmental food supply yet. You've been undereating for quite
a while. It doesn't know that this is a permanent change. The only
way a body can "know" that is after months of good-quality body-
controlled eating.

SYSTEMATIC DESENSITIZATION

A phobia is a fear-induced disability. People who are truly phobic often have great difficulty just getting through the day because
their fear is so powerful and overwhelming. Sometimes people

with eating struggles do, too. Psychologists sometimes treat phobic patients with a therapy known as systematic desensitization. This approach is based on a simple theory—that people who have an inordinate fear of something can increase their tolerance for it by experiencing a series of graded exposures to the thing they fear. For example, a dog-phobic person might first practice talking about dogs or read a book about them. Then she might be brought into a room where there is a dog, out of view and on a leash. Next, the leash, but not the dog, might be brought into view across the room. Then the dog might be brought into view, and led on its leash a bit closer, and so forth. Gradually the person may become at least relatively comfortable with the idea of a dog.

Exercises in Systematic Desensitization

Some people with eating disturbances, especially anorectics, are food phobic. It may be helpful for them to use the principles of systematic desensitization to become less terrified so they can better satisfy their bodies' needs and get on with living. Reading a book like this, about eating more, is a good start. I often advise phobic clients to read the book *without trying any suggestions,* or even focusing on themselves and their own eating problems as they do. Otherwise, they become so frightened that they freeze and can't learn.

After reading it helps to talk with others about eating more. It's very important to hang around with healthy, relaxed, "normal" eaters. (Other eating-disturbed individuals are likely to reinforce your fears.) Discuss the changes you want to make in your eating with a trusted friend, counselor or spouse.

Next, use your imagination to see yourself walking through a buffet line, casually selecting any food that looks good to you. Then see yourself sitting down with friends and eating together, completely relaxed and enjoying yourself, eating until you are satisfied and feeling content.

Practice grocery shopping with your taste buds in mind. Try buying more of the foods you like, and keep a good stock at home. Aim for more variety, perhaps adding some new foods, each time you shop. Take your time buying food, experience the colors, shapes, textures, labels. Have a little fun with it. Do the same when you eat.

When you eat out, don't automatically look for the lowest-fat, lowest-calorie item offered on the menu. Really look at the selections and try to imagine what each would taste like. Consider whether you would enjoy something unusual, or perhaps an old favorite that you haven't had for years. Ask the waiter about it. Then break away and order that.

Here are some self-talk suggestions for combating food phobia:

1. Eating good food when I get hungry is the most natural thing in the world.
2. Eating, by itself, doesn't make people fat; the under-eating/overeating Cycles do.
3. Not eating enough at the right times is at the root of my eating struggles.
4. Eating good food whenever I get hungry is the only way out of my eating disturbance.
5. My body is designed to manage my eating and my weight if I eat enough good food at the right time.
6. Eating well is something everyone does, even the thinnest people.
7. The only way to have a normal relationship with food is to learn to satisfy my hunger consistently.

Since fear of food and fear of losing control of eating behavior, because of enlarged appetites, are reactions to adaptive mechanisms at work, the only true way to moderate them is by changing the food supply—by eating more. But if people are too afraid to eat more because of this phobia, they are truly trapped. Where can they start? At the point of their fear—eating.

Whether you succeed or fail at the Naturally Thin Program for breaking out of food jail depends largely on how you handle your fears. I recommend that you ignore them, and keep your power to decide to do the right and healthful thing, as many of my clients have done. Your fear has kept you locked in an eating disturbance and separated from life in many ways. You don't need to overcome your fear, you need to ignore it and focus on your knowledge, faith and goal to get well. Handling your fear is best done the same way as handling a two-year-old's temper tantrum—ignore it and do what you need to do.

Ignore your fear and pay close attention to the life and healthy eating patterns you desire.

FEAR AND SELF-SABOTAGE

There are several effective ways to rationalize continuing the self-destructive patterns of eating disorders, and fear is behind them all. Rationalization always accompanies self-destructive behaviors because deep down, people feel guilty about them. Rationalizations help ease the guilt. Here's an incomplete list:

1. I'm not going to eat in this self-destructive way forever. Someday I'll stop (after I'm married, after the baby, after the promotion, after the fifth anniversary, after the crisis, etc.).
2. My eating problem is not that bad. There are other bulimics (or whatever) much worse off than I am, and they're doing OK. I feel fine. Well, usually. Sometimes I feel lousy, but then who doesn't?
3. People do other things to their bodies that are much worse than my eating problem, like smoking, drinking, unsafe sex. I don't do any of that stuff. Everybody has a vice.
4. Believe me, being fat is worse in every way than having an eating disturbance. Isn't that why we opt for the crazy eating anyway? The worst, absolute worst thing in the world for me would be to be fat. And I'm not fat (or I'm not as fat as I could be). I have bulimarexia (or whatever), but I'm not fat. If I didn't have an eating disorder I would definitely be fat. My body can never get enough food.

What do you say to yourself to stay in jail? Write it down.

Giving up these excuses for staying in food jail is a big leap toward getting yourself free. Another important step is setting goals for yourself and charting your progress.

GOAL-SETTING IN EATING BEHAVIOR

Sometimes it's helpful to establish specific goals, setting small steps that lead to a bigger, long-term goal. This can help you feel successful while you are in the slow, sometimes tedious process of getting your body in charge of your eating. Although these goals must be individualized, based on your particular disorder, fears, eating patterns, schedule, etc., here are some examples of goal-setting that some of my clients have used with success.

SAMPLE GOAL #1: Get in touch with my hunger feelings by checking with my body every hour, on the hour, throughout the day.

Getting in touch with hunger is essential for everyone, although some will have more trouble with it than others. In order to move toward body-controlled eating, you must learn to recognize your body's requests for fuel, which it usually communicates in several ways. Plain old hunger pangs are rarely missed as signals for food, but shakiness and trouble concentrating may be. Every hour, think about your body's signals—that gurgling in your stomach or dull headache. Make your own list of different ways your body asks for fuel. Call it "empty tank signals." Then watch for them.

SAMPLE GOAL #2: Keep food within reach at all times.

This is an excellent nonthreatening goal because it doesn't address eating at all. Just have food there. Of course, the ultimate point is that it should be eaten, but this goal is a prerequisite to that. Figure out how to have food wherever you are—in a bag lunch or office refrigerator, in your car, in your purse when you shop. Then get it there.

SAMPLE GOAL #3: Eat at least five servings of fruit and vegetables daily.

Always start the actual eating goals with foods that are the least likely to trigger fear. This shouldn't be too terribly frightening—it's about the quality of your eating and variety. Maybe this won't be your weak spot, but it is for many. If you undereat breads, for instance, then try setting a goal there. If you don't drink enough water or abuse diuretics, set specific goals about those things.

SAMPLE GOAL #4: Do not weigh or measure food.

Ex–food controllers usually have withdrawal symptoms when we discuss giving up portion control. This practice is an excellent example of how far we've gone off the deep end in trying to manage our weights by mind-control tactics. Imagine the cavewomen putting their giant meat slabs on a little primitive scale to see how much of the mammoth thigh they should eat! An important part of body-controlled eating involves letting your appetite determine your portions, the way it has been since time began for humans on earth. As long as you are eating enough on a regular basis, and stick with high-quality food, you'll never overeat once you are off the Cycle forever.

SAMPLE GOAL #5: Eliminate poor-quality food.

The key to easy control over food quality is seeing to its availability. It's pretty hard to eat a piece of pecan pie that isn't there. And when ice cream isn't available, there's not a chance that you'll binge on a half gallon. So throw out any foods that don't meet the Real Food criteria—high nutrient value and low fat. And keep it that way. That should keep your eating quality in line with ease, as long as you are eating enough.

SAMPLE GOAL #6: Cut back on laxatives, diuretics or exercise purging tactics.

If you can go cold turkey on these because of your new insights, great. But if you feel threatened about giving up any of these weight-management gimmicks, then proceed in small steps. Try skipping a day of exercise or cutting the daily time back by one-fourth. Laxatives and diuretics that are used daily should be withdrawn slowly so your body has a chance to adjust. Put yourself on a schedule if it helps, gradually eliminating these entrapping behaviors.

Your small goals will be unique to your disorder, your eating patterns, your personality and schedule. Set just a few simple ones at first, say two or three, or even one, if that seems to be all you can handle at first. Don't try to conquer your troubled eating all at once. Any pattern you can identify that should be modified will serve as a worthwhile goal now that you know the direction out of your eating struggles. Goal-setting will also help give you some structure as you begin making changes.

SYMPTOMS OF RECOVERY

Appetite and energy changes are almost immediate for people with eating disturbances who get off the Cycles. These changes reflect the body's need to readapt to the new availability of food and herald your body's changing needs:

1. normalization of hunger and fullness signals (following an initial increase in appetite)
2. cravings for high quality Real Foods
3. increased physical and emotional energy
4. waning preoccupation with eating and food
5. decrease in shame, guilt and anxiety about weight and eating
6. absence of cravings for fatty and sugary foods
7. improved self-esteem and mood
8. increasing interest in new areas of life

RECOVERY TIMETABLE

The Naturally Thin Program gets easier for most people by six to nine months, but the first months are generally the most difficult. Some say this eating program is harder than restrictive undereating (dieting) at this time because of the discipline it takes to eat well and on time all day long. (But remember, there's no pain of hunger and crazy eating behavior to bear, either.) This is when a support group really helps. (We'll discuss organizing a support group later.)

Many people on the Naturally Thin Program report that their eating patterns are relatively stable by six months, but some, especially anorectics, and overweight bulimics often struggle longer. But those who make the adjustment say the changes in eating behavior gradually become a normal part of their lifestyle, and they recover from much of the anxiety that accompanies the "learning to eat enough" phase.

TROUBLESHOOTING

You probably have quite a few questions by now. As you go along, you may have more. Here are some of the most common questions that clients who are recovering from eating disturbances ask me. I hope these cover your questions, too, and perhaps I'll answer some that may come up for you in the future.

QUESTION: OK, I'm a binge eater. And now I'm supposed to eat whenever I get hungry, right? Well, I'm never hungry—at least not before afternoon. Should I go ahead and eat something in the morning anyway?

ANSWER: Often undereaters complain that they never feel hungry because they have trained their bodies to stop sending hunger signals by avoiding food for so long. They have damaged their bodies' normal communication systems. (It's actually adaptive for bodies to acquiesce this way.) Fortunately, this damage can be undone, but not overnight. It takes time and some patience. Even bodies that have survived decades of famine abuse usually begin sending hunger and fullness signals within a few weeks of listening and eating well. And that's the key to getting in touch with your hunger—listen!

I usually recommend that former faminers invite their bodies to signal a need for food by looking at good food that they like (presenting food) every hour or so for the first few weeks, longer if necessary. This way, even if hunger per se isn't experienced, when food looks appealing or appetizing to the person, that's taken as a quiet hunger signal. Gradually, the hunger signals return, and often, when they do, they become strong and distinct. There's no guesswork for hungry naturally thin people.

A bulimic for eleven years, Lana hadn't eaten breakfast since her mother made her eat before school as a child. (Sometimes mothers are right.) The idea of having to learn to eat in the morning was Lana's biggest challenge. She simply was not hungry in the morning—ever.

Lana also experienced a nagging hunger every night, which is typical of morning undereaters. She was used to eating a sizable snack, or a meal, or an all-out binge at that time, and found that she had some trouble sleeping if she skipped it, on the rare occasions when she could. She was willing to try anything because she knew this was a big key to getting off the FeaFam Cycle.

I suggested that Lana make some gradual adjustments to create morning hunger in her reluctant body. First, when she got hungry at eleven or so, she had to increase her intake considerably and keep it up throughout the day. This would help curtail her cravings at night. Then she'd be able to lighten up on her evening snack, only allowing, for example, a piece of fruit or a glass of skim milk after dinner. (Going to bed a little hungry is OK on the Naturally Thin Program because during sleep the body's fuel needs are stable without the stress of physical activity.) If this change didn't make breakfast more appealing, she could always eliminate the evening snack altogether once her daytime eating became adequate. Remember, she was willing to try anything until she found something that worked.

Well, she didn't have to go to extremes. Once Lana began to eat more during the day, she was amazed that her evening cravings and bingeing stopped soon after! She found she was able to cut back on, and then eliminate, after-dinner eating without much trouble. When she did, she began to wake up a little hungry.

These changes seemed like a miracle to Lana. She was surprised, as many people breaking out of food jail are, at how quickly her body responded, and at its mysterious ability to normalize her appetite in response to her new eating choices. She had been afraid of eating more at first, but her fear quickly turned to relief. Lana has been completely free of bulimia and the FeaFam Cycle symptoms for four years.

QUESTION: I'm a compulsive overeater and I have just the opposite problem—I'm always hungry! What should I do—eat all day long?

ANSWER: Oddly, this is the other most common complaint where hunger signals are concerned. Either undereaters are never hungry or they are always hungry! Obviously, going hungry is very confusing to bodies!

Another way the body adapts to chronic eating avoidance is chronic hunger signals. This can make a dieter extremely anxious about her appetite and afraid of turning the eating controls over to her body. It seems as if her body is determined to have her eating twenty-four hours a day nonstop!

In the transition phase of getting off the Cycles, most ex-faminers, even the ones who initially "never feel hungry," have to learn to eat adequate amounts of good food often. This is because they have some make-up eating to do as their bodies compensate for undereating. The last feast is the most frightening phase of recovery for many. Fortunately, it doesn't last very long for most. Usually by the third week, the appetite diminishes and the cravings change to herald readaptation—the body's readjustment to the new availability of food.

So if you're hungry "all the time" at the beginning, don't fight it—eat! The tendency for most ex-faminers is to continue to control portions at the beginning especially, but that will only keep you on the Cycle, so don't do it if you can take the plunge. Let go. Eat Real Food until you are satisfied every time you get hungry. Be especially careful to eat to your satisfaction point early in the day because eating well at this time has a normalizing effect on your appetite later in the day, when make-up cravings are most common. The sooner you let go and give in to your hunger each time, the sooner your appetite and body can get back to normal.

QUESTION: I used to be anorectic, but I've developed bulimia in the last year. I never eat breakfast. In fact, I feel a little nauseated first thing in the morning. Why is that? Will it interfere with my getting off the Cycle?

ANSWER: Slight early-morning nausea or disinterest in food is so common that I consider it normal, even for some naturally thin people. Unfortunately, though, this tendency predisposes a person to the Feast or Famine Cycle because, by the time these underfed people are hungry, often food is unavailable. Breakfast skippers experience daily famines, and if they are famine sensitive, they usually experience cravings and do make-up eating in the afternoon and/or evening to compensate, perhaps with loss of control.

Ex-dieters who don't feel especially like eating right away in the morning usually feel slightly hungry within thirty minutes or an hour, if they are listening. Of course, if they are rushing around trying to get the kids off to school and get ready for work or school, they are probably not listening. And their bodies may not be talking anymore, either. This is a good example of how a person, over time, gets out of touch with her body's fuel needs. Physical activity without fuel is a serious famine situation that must be, and can only be, prevented by making your body's fuel needs a priority.

If you are not a first-thing-in-the-morning eater, you will have to listen very carefully for those first hunger hints. Then, if you are ready, have something light and palatable, like a muffin and juice. This tells your body that food is available and invites it to send fuel-need signals. If you will not be home when the hunger hits (usually within an hour or two), you must pack Real Food and take it with you. Even if you are planning a midmorning meal out, take food with you. It is unlikely that your hunger and your brunch date will coincide perfectly. Always be prepared to eat when hunger strikes.

QUESTION: Carrying food around all day sounds pretty inconvenient. Will I have to take food with me for the rest of my life?

ANSWER: Probably. I still do, and it has kept me thin and out of food jail for over ten years. I admit it is a bit inconvenient, but then, my crazy eating habits were worse for me by far.

As you get to know your body better, you won't have to guess so often about how much and what foods to take with you. Also, as your body readapts to this new food supply, it will get on a schedule of sorts. Your hunger signals will come generally about the same time every day (unless your activity level changes), so planning your meals will get easier.

You don't have to pack everything, either. I rely on a grocery store deli section near my office for some meals throughout the day. Also, some fast-food restaurants are offering higher-quality Real Foods now. Check out their nutrition information and keep track of the best-quality foods they offer. And remember, eating something when you're hungry is always better than going hungry. So if you're stuck in a situation with nothing better to eat than a fast-food burger, eat it. But learn the lesson and prepare better for your hunger in the future. Hamburgers just aren't good enough for your body, right?

QUESTION: What kinds of foods can I carry with me?

ANSWER: Sandwiches are designed for packing, and the possibilities are unlimited. Make an effort to use a variety of whole-grain breads and quality fillings. The Earl of Sandwich, who designed the portable meal, must have been naturally thin!

By the way, normal sandwiches are made with two slices of bread (yes, that's two whole slices) with something in between. Bread, we have recently "learned," is a staple of a healthful diet, so don't try to limit your bread intake anymore. And fillings choices can stretch your creativity—veggies, peanut butter and fruit, lean meats or dairy products. But don't just think about it! Eat some sandwiches.

Fruits are very portable. If you're worried about food spoiling, buy a small cooler to keep with you. Muffins and bagels are easy to transport. Check labels if you are unsure about the quality of the ingredients. Nuts and seeds, including trail mixes, are made for packing. (Watch the fat in the nuts and seeds, though, and keep these for more occasional use, say, once or twice a week.) Raw vegetables can be packed with dip, if you have a cooler, and lower-fat cheeses and whole-grain, low-fat crackers are quite portable, too.

Use your imagination and your appetite and make a list of your own. Don't focus on low-calorie foods! Instead, pack the best-quality Real Foods you can find. Your job is to maximize, not minimize, eating quality calories within your body's fuel-need signals. A common mistake for undereaters is to pack foods that are unsubstantial—that don't have enough good calories to really satisfy their hunger. This tendency, of course, comes from years of trying to eat less. But you're not trying to eat less anymore, right?

Betsy came for coaching after struggling with bulimarexia for almost three years. She immediately understood the Feast or Famine Cycle and agreed that she needed to stop starving herself. Determined to get back in touch with her hunger, Betsy promised to start eating.

Two months later Betsy called me, very discouraged. She was eating every time she felt hungry, but still had some binge/purge episodes that frightened her back into starving herself. It was clear that she was not off the FeaFam Cycle.

As we went over her eating, I knew what was wrong. Betsy was eating in response to her hunger all right, but only very small amounts of food. I call this "medicating hunger." For example, she'd have a small carton of sugar-free, fat-free yogurt and black coffee for breakfast. Then, when she got hungry at about nine-thirty, she'd have an orange or half a bagel. Lunch was a cup of vegetable soup. No crackers, no sandwich, no milk. The rest of the day followed the same pattern until about eight o'clock at night. Then Betsy would begin to get really hungry and find herself losing control at times.

Betsy had to stop medicating her hunger and start really satisfying it. This fact flew in the face of her fear of gaining weight, but she was ready to try. And she did. By doubling and tripling her food intake, Betsy was completely free of her eating troubles six weeks later.

QUESTION: I just can't eat anytime I feel hungry at my job. Any suggestions?

ANSWER: Most jobs allow for breaks between meals, either formal or informal. In fact, employers have a legal responsibility to provide break time to workers, besides the traditional mealtimes. These breaks are usually flexible with most employers and can be taken when you get hungry. If not, you may have to be creative in order to eat on time at work.

Very quick (two-minute) powder room breaks can be slipped in for a mini-meal. Usually beverages are not forbidden in the work environment and you can use a high-nutrient powder mix in milk or juice for secret nutrient consumption. Most employers are very cooperative and will make some adjustments if you just ask.

Flora is a critical care nurse, and a self-diagnosed compulsive overeater (bulimic), about sixty pounds overweight. She described her eight-hour shift, full of physical activity and a lot of stress. She said it was impossible for her to eat at all during her shift, except on an occasional "slow" night. She always experienced powerful cravings for sweets and fatty foods after work, and she was relieved to find that these cravings had to do with her serious undereating at work. She asked if it was possible for her to get off the Feast or Famine Cycle in light of the eating limitations at her job.

It was certainly obvious to me why Flora was so over-weight, in light of her high physical activity level and serious undereating! She had severe famines almost daily built right into her job. (A severe famine is very restricted food availability plus high physical output.)

As I explored possible solutions to her poor food availability on the job, it became obvious that there simply weren't any feasible ways to improve it enough to allow her to get off the Cycle. With emergencies and the nearly constant demands of a critical care unit, Flora simply could not integrate eating well or often enough into her shift schedule to break her body's adaptive symptoms. I suggested that she consider transferring into another area of nursing for the sake of her health. This may sound extreme, but in her particular job situation Flora's chances for getting her eating patterns back to normal were just about zero.

QUESTION: A food addict, I've been trying this body-controlled eating for about two weeks. I still crave sweets. Why?

ANSWER: Cravings generally reflect the body's needs. If you crave high-sugar foods that are typically low in nutrient value, your body needs the fat these foods can supply. Remember, your body's need for fat is a result of the famines it has experienced during your diets or undereating periods. Biochemicals control these cravings and you want biochemical adjustments to be made in your body when you turn the eating controls over to it. In other words, when the famines stop, these cravings will change.

As you continue to eat well whenever you are hungry, your body will gradually sense the change in the availability of food and your cravings will shift to leaner, more healthful foods. Your body will need a new type of food in this plentiful environment because it will have different priorities. The need for excess fat and the five adaptive mechanisms that promote it will be eliminated. The need for optimal nutrition will take its place. Sweets (and fatty foods) are not particularly appealing to the person who is not on the Cycle.

If you have just lost some weight, or you have been dieting recently, the cravings for Pleasure Foods may continue for a few months. Be careful, though, because continued cravings for sweets and fats are also symptoms of staying on the Cycle. If these cravings continue past the first few weeks, you may *not* be off the Cycle. In other words, you may not be eating enough Real Food on time to satisfy your body.

> A self-proclaimed chocaholic and bulimarectic, Louise laughed out loud when I told her she would stop craving sweets once she was off the FeaFam Cycle. She said she wasn't born with a silver spoon in her mouth, she was born with a chocolate one! It was absolutely inconceivable to her that she could ever get through a day without her chocolate fix. She hadn't gone a day without chocolate for fifteen years, even when she was anorectic! Chocolate was an essential part of her life.
>
> During her third week Louise called me. She was in shock, she said. It couldn't be true, but it was true and it was her body! She had not had any chocolate for five days, and although she had some in her freezer, she absolutely didn't want any! Louise laughed again—and cried—from relief.

QUESTION: I don't know when I'm hungry and I'm never full. I'm nineteen and I've been anorectic for four years. Why?

ANSWER: Many people who have violated their bodies' hunger signals for a long time complain about difficulties with hunger and fullness sensations. Again, these troubles are a result of the long-term body abuse of going hungry much of the time, and then, for most, overeating to compensate.

Naturally thin people generally know when they are hungry, what they are hungry for and when to stop eating. This is because their bodies are in charge of their eating and their bodies' fuel-need and -full signals are perfectly intact.

It takes time to reestablish the lines of communication between the self-starver and her body—time and plenty of good food. So be patient, but know that your body can do this.

For those who have great difficulty with these signals, I suggest that they take hourly breaks in their day to consciously check for hunger. Sometimes it's helpful to look at good food at these times. If it looks appealing, that's hunger. And when they are eating, it usually helps them get in touch with fullness by pausing every now and then during the meal.

Although this process sounds tedious, it usually doesn't take too long for those who need extra help in this area. Bodies, I have found, are remarkably forgiving once you offer them the attention and care they deserve.

QUESTION: I'm bulimic. I've been doing the Naturally Thin Program for six weeks, and I still overeat at supper now and then. What's wrong?

ANSWER: Overeating is an adaptive symptom of the Cycle, and if you still have the urge to do it, your body still needs fat. You have to find out why. Either you are still recovering from your last famine and your body isn't ready to level off because of the severity or length of that famine, or you are still sometimes famining (undereating) now.

Most often people breaking out of food jail who weren't dieting strictly and had been at a relatively stable weight before they began the program have stopped experiencing the urge to overeat by six weeks, some by two. If you didn't experience a recent weight loss or "successful" diet, you are probably still on the Cycle. That means you are still undereating or eating poor-quality food at times, which keeps the adaptive urge to overeat going. Bodies don't overeat for no reason. You need to find the famine in your current eating schedule.

"Finding the famine" helps ex-faminers understand the link between their undereating or poor food quality and their overeating. Usually missed meals occur at two critical times during the day: midmorning and late afternoon. Lousy, nutrient-poor food may slip into your diet, so check your diet for food quality, too. Sometimes increasing your activity level without keeping up with your extra energy needs can create a famine.

Famine-sensitive people need to eat good food often. Three meals a day isn't usually often enough, and I've found that women in general, and sometimes men too, need at least five quality meals a day. Because of this, you should plan to eat at least three meals by about one o'clock in the afternoon, if you're on a regular nine-to-five work routine. This means, breakfast as soon as possible after waking, brunch between nine-thirty and eleven and lunch by one or so. Of course, if you have a different day/night schedule, you can adjust those guidelines according to your wake-up time.

These times are only guidelines, based on observations of what seems to work best for most people in recovery. Again, don't watch the clock but stay tuned to your body. We offer this schedule because most people with eating problems have absolutely no idea of what to expect from their bodies once they start eating more normally, and it helps to know what other people usually experience.

Besides breakfast, the most commonly missed "mealtime" is late afternoon. Like breakfast time, late afternoon is usually a very busy time when eating is inconvenient if not impossible. But people who want to straighten out their eating have to make eating well at this time a priority because it is critical to recovery. This is the very best time to spoil your dinner and occasionally, if you have done a great job of eating on time all day long, you may not even want much dinner!

QUESTION: You keep talking about eating often enough. I'm eating every hour and a half to two hours because that's how often I'm hungry! Is this normal?

ANSWER: Yes. Naturally thin people, especially women, sometimes eat that frequently, especially early in the day when their activity levels are highest. This translates to four meals by 1 P.M. or so.

If you are eating that often all day long, it is possible that your diet is too light: too low in calories, protein and/or fat. High-carbohydrate diets are very popular now, but sometimes people try to cut way down on proteins and cut out fats and wind up feeling unsatisfied too much of the day. Adequate protein foods in your diet, especially early in the day, can help keep you satisfied longer so you don't have to eat as frequently. And fats (vegetable fats are best) also burn more slowly, keeping your appetite satisfied longer. A low-fat diet doesn't mean a no-fat diet. Fats play an important role in a healthy, balanced diet and you need to integrate them sparingly and wisely.

HOW A VERY LOW FAT DIET CAN LEAD TO EATING DISTURBANCES

Candace found out from her doctor that her cholesterol level was too high. She advised her to cut down on dietary fat and gave her an article that explained how to do it. Candace was very motivated because there was heart disease in her family. So fat grams became the focus of her eating choices. She was slightly overweight and had never had an eating problem.

Candace switched from eggs and buttered toast to that special no-fat cereal and skim milk. She also had fruit for breakfast and between meals. So far so good—zero grams of fat. Then she passed up the cream-based soups she loved and had vegetables swimming in low-fat chicken broth. Pretty tasty too, as she found her hunger rather intense. With her new light soup, Candace chose a low-fat pasta dish or half a sandwich filled with very low fat meats, tuna or vegetables. Delicious. She started using skim milk in her coffee and never, ever touched butter. The choices for supper were endless: pasta in low-fat tomato sauce, baked potatoes with low-fat yogurt on top, stir-fry low-fat anything (no oil) with rice. Doesn't this sound healthy? You bet it does.

But after about a week of following this low-fat regimen, Candace found herself eating a whole bowl of potato chips at a friend's house. This shocked her. She almost never even wanted potato chips, and now, when she knew she should avoid them, she ate a whole bag!

Two days later Candace woke up in the middle of the night absolutely starving. She snuck down to the kitchen and ate her teenage son's leftover cheeseburger—cold! Something was wrong. This just wasn't like her. Her eating seemed to be out of control.

Low-fat diets can set people up for the Feast or Famine Cycle. When you take most or all of the fat out of a diet the calories drop rather dramatically. The body picks up on this drop and perceives it as a famine. And voilà, the adaptive responses are set in motion. If people who go on low-fat diets don't realize this and learn to pay attention to their hunger, they'll start Cycling as a result.

When you eat a lower-fat diet, you need to eat more food, sometimes more often. The lighter food you eat won't last as long in your digestive tract, so you'll get hungry more often and naturally need to eat more often too, in order to prevent a famine. So eat low-fat, but stay tuned to your body. It knows what it needs and will tell you if you keep listening.

TIMETABLE FOR BREAKING OUT OF FOOD JAIL

Many clients ask me to advise them how long it will take them to get back to normal eating. As the case studies show, each person is unique, with a distinct food problem. Although there are patterns in the disturbances, there are many variables as well. What I can say with confidence is this: Complete recovery usually takes years. Eating patterns always normalize first, sometimes within weeks, but weight shifts always take longer, often years to complete. There are exceptions, and they are always surprising.

The reason that the restoration of normal eating patterns, and especially weight, is such a long process is simple and revealing: bodies are not equipped to make quick adjustments to changes in the food supply. In fact, it is our presumption of the body's ability to make such hasty adaptations that has gotten us into such deep diet trouble in the first place. We have to put these erroneous prejudices aside if we are ever going to make serious progress in this field of healthy eating and weight management.

CHAPTER 6

Breaking Free to a New Body Image

SELF-IMPOSED UNDEREATING AND BODY-IMAGE DISTORTION go together. People who chronically or intermittently undereat in an effort to control weight almost always suffer from unrealistic, and sometimes bizarre, perceptions of their own body size. They typically see their bodies as very much larger, heavier and bulkier than they really are. Tragically, this phenomenon promotes their commitment to undereating, the hallmark of eating disturbances.

An opposite type of body-image distortion sometimes occurs among overweight people who have just recently gained a significant amount of weight and more rarely in people with long-term obesity. This distortion can also be found among ex-dieters who have learned body-controlled eating but have not lost their excess weight yet. These people see themselves as thinner, and sometimes *much* thinner, than they really are. They are shocked, they say, when they catch glimpses of themselves in storefront windows. They don't recognize the heavy body they see as their own.

Do these distortions of reality serve some adaptive function, or are they examples of the body/mind connection going completely haywire? Perhaps denial of emaciation that anorectics and some bulimics experience has some protective aspect that we don't know about. Or maybe it's a function of the emaciation itself—a result of biochemical imbalance from starvation. Or both.

Anorectics' insistence that they are still fat when they are extremely thin appears to protect them from their fear of losing control with food. If they admit the truth—that they are really thin, even too thin, it's like a green light to loosen up on their rigid eating controls. This is terrifying for people who have successfully barricaded themselves against their own survival instincts concerning food. They are trapped by their fear of losing control, and no degree of thinness is going to lead them from their self-imposed prison. They do not want to be free. They are afraid of freedom because they are convinced that it will positively lead to overweight.

Melissa had just turned fourteen when she was hospitalized for "tests." She had been losing weight steadily since the beginning of the school year eight months before. But it was her ferocious insistence that she was getting fatter that concerned her parents the most. She was down to 105 pounds on a five-foot five-inch frame.

For a few days Melissa refused almost all food. Her nurse never commented or criticized her, but brought her trays in and took them out. Melissa began to talk to her and open up a bit. One evening this nurse brought her dinner tray and noticed Melissa looking down at her bare thighs. "My legs are so huge," she complained. "Aren't they enormous?" "Do you want me to be honest?" the nurse replied. "Yes, tell me the truth. They're huge and gross, aren't they?" Melissa said. "No, they're not," said the nurse. "Your legs are thin. They're very thin. You just can't see it. I'm telling you the truth."

Although she argued with the nurse, Melissa gradually began to eat more after that, and slowly gained back the weight she'd lost and a bit more. She eventually leveled off at a higher and healthier weight. Unlike severe anorectics, Melissa was still open to reality regarding her body.

Staying open to reason is dangerous to most anorectics and people with other types of eating problems because it could lead to letting their guard down. This is exactly what happened to Melissa, and it broke her self-imposed famine and got her started eating more. Fortunately, she was not very far down the anorectic road and still had a chance to escape from food jail. She was able to turn back to healthy eating and a more normal body image without the major effort that is usually necessary.

FEAR, ANXIETY, STRESS AND BODY-IMAGE DISTORTION

Fear, anxiety and stress normally cause an adaptive depression of the appetite. This effect is physiological and adaptive because our chronic digestive needs are a lower survival priority than coping with danger or potential danger. Consequently, fear, anxiety and stress promote famines—adaptive famines, but famines nonetheless.

Just five weeks before her younger sister, the baby of the family, died from cancer, Alice found out about it. It seemed unbelievable to her. Alice shared the hospital vigils with her brother and an aunt, but felt especially committed to her sister. They had had a very difficult relationship and Alice felt guilty and remorseful about things she had said and done. Somehow she felt responsible for her sister.

For the first time in her life Alice had trouble eating. She simply had no appetite. She was actually nauseated at times and couldn't bring herself to eat anything. Occasionally, she'd have a cookie or a donut, but that was about it. By the time the funeral was over and all the thank-you notes mailed, Alice had lost over fifteen pounds.

When she came to me for coaching, Alice had gained nearly thirty pounds over the following year. She was completely perplexed about this because she'd never had a weight problem before.

When people are stressed, excited or emotionally upset, their normal hunger signals often get blocked out. By the time they calm down, they have a famine to recover from, with cravings and the tendency to binge. This is how these emotions can promote weight gain.

The fear of weight gain is, in itself, an enormous stress for many people. And it is universal in the eating disturbed. This fear can become a chronic (anorexia) or intermittent (bulimia, compulsive overeating, food addiction, etc.) appetite suppressant in them. And it is one reason individuals with eating disorders always report trouble with their hunger signals. They are out of touch with their need for food in part because their fear has become a threat to their emotional safety. Part of this loss of appetite is frank denial (I don't want to be hungry so I'm not), but some is definitely physiological—the suppressant effect of fear, anxiety and stress on the appetite center.

In the eating disturbed, typically, as the body becomes smaller, the mind's perception of body size grows, perhaps to compensate for the threat of starvation. This is the strangest paradox of eating disturbances.

Here's another irony. In most eating-disturbed individuals, the distortion of their body image goes in the direction of their fear. The object of their obsessive fear and undereating—overweight—is fantasized into reality by their minds. This is an amazing phenomenon. It is their fear of gaining weight that hooks undereaters in the first place, and then, as they move further and further away from the condition they fear, they create that same condition by distorting their body size in their minds. It's wild. I have been there myself and I have counseled many others in this condition.

The distortion of body image in fearful undereaters fuels their determination to avoid food. They create or exaggerate their weight problems in order to stay afraid enough to continue to resist one of the most powerful biological urges in human beings—to satisfy hunger by eating food. And the reverse is true, too. Undereating for weight control itself seems to promote a distortion in perceived body size. These distortions are true for all anorectics, most bulimics and many undereating dieters as well.

UNREALISTIC BODY-IMAGE MESSAGES

We all know that the model-thin standard for American women has caused a lot of pain and struggle for many of us, whether or not we have actual eating disorders. I'm not going to rehash this dismal cause/effect relationship because others have done this well. Let me simply remind you that you are undoubtedly under the influence of the ultra-light body expectations of our thinness-crazed culture. There is almost no way to escape them. But I know there are ways to do serious damage to these messages and the insidious influence they have on us.

The tactics that follow are deprogramming devices, to be practiced routinely (and gladly) in order to enjoy maximum benefits. Deprogramming unrealistic body-image ideals that have been drilled into one's mind for years, or decades, does not come quickly. Even if body weight normalizes, and the eating disturbance is conquered, body-image conflicts usually continue indefinitely, although to a lesser degree.

Renoir's Women

Pierre-Auguste Renoir, a French Impressionist painter during the latter nineteenth and early twentieth centuries, used intense color and contouring. He painted mostly sensual scenes, parties of young handsome people drinking and dancing, and lovely children in rich clothing and settings. But especially, Renoir had a painter's eye for beautiful women.

For our purposes the most essential fact about Renoir's women was that they were quite fat by our standards. Yet their poses do not give a hint of any concern whatever with their broad, round hips or ample tummies and thighs. In fact, they all look very content and even quietly proud to be standing or sitting there with plenty of padding everywhere. And what's so interesting about looking at these wonderful paintings is this: you discover that these women are beautiful, and their voluptuous bodies are beautiful, too!

What's the point? Your *attitude* toward your body can make a big difference in how you *look* to others and how you *feel* about yourself.

And one more thing: Renoir's women illustrate the fact that the standard for ideal body size is arbitrary and changing. We can set our own standard, based on what we're comfortable with and what works for our individual bodies. This may take some effort, but may be more practical in the long run than endlessly trying to squeeze into sizes for which we are not designed.

BODY-IMAGE COPING TACTIC #1:

1. Buy or borrow a book of Renoir's paintings.
2. Study the paintings of women.
3. Think about the lives of those women, how at peace they seem with their bodies.
4. Consider your body in the context of Renoir's time.
5. Take a deep breath.
6. Smile.
7. Repeat as needed.

COURAGE CENTER

*"My stomach is so big I can't stand it. I can't get rid of it. I
hate it. I absolutely hate it. And my thighs—they are so fat that
they rub together when I walk. I absolutely hate that feeling. I
can't wear short skirts. I can't fit into my size sevens anymore.
My stomach is just, well, look at it. Isn't it sticking out like a
pregnant woman? That's what it looks like—pregnant. Oh,
God, what am I going to do?"*

*Gretchen was in such obvious pain as she spoke that she
almost cried. She looked anxious and depressed as she described her body's trouble spots. Gretchen was five feet six
inches tall and weighed 135 pounds. She had weighed 122
two years before. I recommended that Gretchen visit Courage
Center.*

Located in Golden Valley, Minnesota, Courage Center is a place
for people who need very extensive rehabilitation, mostly for injuries. There children hurt in farm accidents learn to use artificial
arms and legs. Teens with brain injuries learn to talk again or use
other ways of communicating. And there are many determined
people at Courage Center with spinal cord injuries, some with
lower body paralysis who must learn to get along without the use
of their legs—no movement, no feeling left. And there are quadri-
plegics—usually young people who have broken their necks, losing control of their whole bodies, except the head. These patients
must adopt a wheelchair for locomotion and need a companion
for most basic activities of daily living. And there are stroke victims
and kids with cerebral palsy. The list is long.

This visit was not to shame Gretchen. It was to jolt her into a
new perspective. Sometimes we need that.

BODY-IMAGE COPING TACTIC #2:

1. Make a list of everyone you know about who is struggling
   with a physical problem.
2. Think of each individual and his/her problem.
3. Consider your own physical strengths.
4. Write down your body's capabilities. List everything, even
   routine things you take for granted, like taking a shower.

5. Say, "I appreciate my body and all the wonderful things it can do."
6. Say it again, louder.
7. Repeat anytime a rash of self-pity appears.

TAKE THIS SIZE AND SHOVE IT

In general, women are obsessive about the sizes they wear. Fitting into a certain size can make or break the day. "Oh, it fits! It actually fits—a ten! I can't believe it! A ten, a ten. This is wonderful!" And growing out of a size is catastrophic, causing protracted depression and social isolation. "No, I can't go to the wedding. I know he's my son, but I'm back in a sixteen."

What if there were no sizes? (It will be like this in heaven.) What if we just put on big wraparounds and never even knew if we were size two, size twelve or size twenty? What would a no-size wardrobe and lifestyle be like? I'll tell you: it would be far more sane for some of us than the world we live in now.

BODY-IMAGE COPING TACTIC #3:

1. Take all of the clothes in your closet that are too small (unless you are pregnant) and put them in boxes.
2. Give them to the Salvation Army or the Goodwill.
3. Get a permanent marking pen.
4. Mark all your clothes that fit you well the size you want to be.
5. Enjoy.

IF THE CLOTHES FIT, WEAR 'EM

Clothes are made for the body, not the other way around. We're tempted to try to fit our bodies into certain clothing sizes, but wouldn't it be better to try to find clothes that are attractive and really fit comfortably?

When my daughter, Genevieve, went through a rather dramatic growth spurt during her fourteenth year, she fairly flew through three sizes in nine months. One autumn she was squarely in a seven and by spring the tens and twelves were feeling uncomfortable to her. Did she diet? Did she desperately try to exercise her way back to her smaller-sized clothes? She did not.

The next time we shopped Genevieve picked the next larger size and one size bigger than that to try on. She didn't pay any attention to the numbers on the clothes. She was looking for her style in a comfortable fit. Her approach was, "Hey, my body's all right, I just have to find the clothes that are right for my body." Comfort was her top goal, along with looking attractive. She paid no attention to the sizes she'd outgrown and has no prejudices about the size she "should" be. Her attitude is: the size I am is the right size for me.

BODY-IMAGE COPING TACTIC #4:

1. When you shop for clothes, try on a larger size than you usually wear.
2. Keep comfort in mind as a top priority when choosing clothes.
3. If you try on something that's too small, remind yourself, My body's right, these clothes are wrong.
4. Always remember: clothes are made for the body, not the other way around.

SELF-ACCEPTANCE AND FAT TOLERANCE

I read a lot these days about fat acceptance. Accept your fat, love your fat. If you're fat, just love yourself unreservedly and it'll be OK, right? I don't think it's quite that simple.

This first formula is designed to compensate for fat rejection. People who are fat (or think they are) tend to reject the fat and then reject themselves as well. This sad state of affairs is a consequence of the power of The Thin Ideal in our country.

Is there a more realistic and helpful approach to this mix-up between body size and self-esteem? Yes, and the key lies in separating them as much as possible. Our body size is not who we are. Got that? It must be tolerated if it doesn't fit our ideal, and statistics show that for most of us it doesn't. Most of us are disappointed with our figures at best, and horrified at worst, so it's a good idea for all of us to learn body tolerance.

But the self, which is a very different thing from the body, will do much better with a more affirmative approach—grace and acceptance. To advise someone who thinks she is overweight to accept or embrace her condition is expecting too much. But as you learn to tolerate your physical imperfections, you can work toward greater self-acceptance.

You learn that you aren't entirely to blame for your physical imperfection, and that your body problems are not negative reflections on you and who you are. You can enjoy your personal attributes and tackle your weaknesses with greater success without beating yourself up for not being thin enough. And your chances of enjoying yourself and succeeding in other areas of life are maximized by embracing who you are and learning to put up with disappointing realities.

So tolerate the aspects of your body that you don't like, and work at accepting and developing your self.

BODY-IMAGE COPING TACTIC #5:

1. List five features you like about your body. (Yes, you can.) More if possible.
2. List five features you like about yourself or other people say they like about you.
3. Hang these lists wherever you spend time and read them daily.
4. List five things you would like to change about your body—any feature, height, hair color, etc.
5. Cross off anything on the list that isn't possible to change. These things are to be tolerated.
6. List five features you would like to change about yourself.
7. Cross off anything on the list that isn't possible.
8. Make one doable goal for improving your body and one doable goal for improving yourself.
9. Do them.

AN EXERCISE IN REGRESSION

Some gifts that come with maturity make us prone to certain kinds of suffering, such as from standards, comparisons and ideals of beauty. By contrast, most children are mysteriously free of the self-scrutiny that comes with trying to measure up to some cultural standard, particularly standards of beauty, and are to be envied for this freedom. We who submit to the merciless taskmaster called The Thin Ideal know the discouragement and unending struggle that our too-conscious minds must endure.

The immaturity of childhood protects little ones in many ways from a sometimes too-acute awareness that grown-ups must live with. Children are quite out of touch with the past, with the future, with the rigid order of things that adults must cope with daily. Little kids live in a world sublimely subjective and somewhat disassociated from adult reality. This is the bliss of their innocence.

You were once there, before the poisonous "you must be very thin to be acceptable" message reached you. Why not disengage yourself from these powerful maxims regarding body size and become more like the little child you once were—free of these musts and shoulds? Is it possible to get away from this indoctrination? We've almost been programmed like cult members when it comes to our attitudes about thinness. How can we be deprogrammed? Slowly, gradually and probably never thoroughly.

BODY-IMAGE COPING TACTIC #6:

1. Like a kid, ignore your bathroom scale.
2. Watch little kids when you get the chance—observe their nonchalance about their bodies, their physical joy. Imitate them.
3. Kids don't study fashion magazines or take weight-loss commercials seriously. Follow their example.
4. To bring you back to that carefree time in your life before body standards, run through a sprinkler, play with squirt guns or do something else that children do for thrills.

MIRROR, MIRROR ON THE WALL

The Amish have a valuable rule designed to curtail vanity and pride: the use of mirrors is prohibited altogether. I think this is a very good idea for many reasons besides preventing vanity and pride. Great big mirrors, perfected reflectors of the twentieth century, are a menace to all who struggle with eating problems. They tell the whole story—every flaw, every bulge and imperfection glares back at us in a full-length mirror. We are almost always disappointed with what we see, and often moved to set our determination to eat less several notches higher.

What we see in a big mirror, if we suffer from the body-image distortion typical of eating-disturbed people, is not what's really there anyway, so why look at all? Because we need to look. We want reassurance. Either we want to be reassured about just how bad we look or how good, if we're in a "successful phase" of our eating control.

But what does this mirror-gazing bring? Reminders of our body consciousness, which we already have in excess. And it brings fear—more fear of looking too big. And frustration, and pain, and irrational thinking, and tunnel vision, and insecurity, and perhaps despair. But we do it because we need to look. We want reassurance. We never stop to think that the reassurance is rarely there, and it is never there for some and never will be.

BODY-IMAGE COPING TACTIC #7:

1. Cover all the mirrors in your house below the face level. Yes you can, for at least a day.
2. Cover all your full-length mirrors entirely.
3. As much as possible, avoid catching glimpses of yourself in store windows and other public reflecting materials.
4. Take these sabbaticals from your physical reflection for longer periods, if you can, say, up to a week.
5. How does it feel to be mirror-free?
6. Write down your thoughts and feelings about having mirrors in your life, out of your life. Decide if you want them in.

THE SCALE AND I

People who cope with disturbed eating have a love/hate relationship with their bathroom scales.

Tom, a bodybuilder with anorexia, compulsively weighed himself six to twenty times a day. He had a professional medical scale, guaranteed accurate to within an ounce, and he was saving for a digital readout scale and had been very excited when a company came out with a travel scale. It was hard for Tom to go even a few hours without knowing what he weighed.

Lois couldn't step on a scale to save her life. She was absolutely petrified of weighing herself or of being weighed by someone else. She refused to be weighed at the doctor's office and actually changed doctors when one insisted on knowing her weight. Lois had developed this aversion to scales when her bulimia followed four years of anorexia.

What power this little instrument wields! I have found that a person's relationship with the scale often reflects her diagnosis with amazing accuracy. The compulsive weighing and the phobic avoidance both occur in people with anorexia, bulimia, bulimarexia, food addiction and compulsive overeating. Rarely do I find an individual with an eating disturbance who is neutral about scales.

BODY-IMAGE COPING TACTIC #8:

1. Throw your scale away. In the garbage. Yes you can.
2. Do you like scale-free living?
3. Keep working on becoming scale-free by resisting the urge to weigh yourself and refusing to be weighed (unless medically necessary).
4. Find out what your weight is in stones (the British and Canadian unit).
5. Use this number and unit when you are asked what you weigh. How does it feel?
6. Adjust your scale, if you must use one, to ten or twenty pounds lighter. Keep it there. Are your days going better?
7. Tape the weight you want to be over the dial. Do you feel better now?

HOLDING YOURSELF UP

My mother used to remind me to sit up straight quite often because I have a natural tendency to slump. She'd say, "Jeanie, straighten up. Pretend there's a string tied to your breastbone that's hanging from the ceiling. Relax your shoulders and push your chest out. Be proud you're a girl!" Later, when my weight became my number-one priority, she added, "You can look ten pounds thinner just by sitting up straight."

And she was right. I have found that good posture is a valuable habit to cultivate for many reasons, including improved appearance. It's good for your attitude, both toward the world and toward yourself. Any doctor will share with you the many advantages of good posture for your spine, circulation, digestion and breathing. But what has this got to do with eating problems?

Disturbed eating behavior is extremely stressful to the body. It often pushes the adaptive potential of the body to the limits, wearing it down both structurally and physiologically. It takes time, and many healthful habits, to restore it to its best. Sitting, standing, walking and lying with your back straight, relaxed and aligned are some important habits that contribute to becoming whole again. And good posture does make you look better.

BODY-IMAGE COPING TACTIC #9:

1. Tie a string to your top buttonhole to remind you to "hang from the ceiling."
2. Practice sitting and walking tall—maximizing your height—when you are exercising.
3. Make sure the main chair you use is posture friendly. Find a new one if it's not.
4. Check your main work area at home and office for organizational changes you can make to lighten the stress on your back.
5. Find a firm little pillow to use at the small of your back when you are sitting for longer periods.
6. Is this a problem area for you? See a health professional who can recommend exercises to strengthen weak posture muscles (abdomen and lower back especially).
7. Like a good mother, remind yourself to straighten up by placing a few love notes in places where you tend to slip.
8. Remember that the posture your body assumes often reflects your "posture" toward life.

BODY-IMAGE CONVERSION

Since self-imposed undereating is such a big factor in body-image distortion, it's the place to start changing if you want to gain a healthy body image. The controlled undereating that inspires all the adaptive responses that make up the symptoms of eating disturbances has to stop. The Feast or Famine Cycle and its variations has to be eliminated. Otherwise, all the body affirmations in the world aren't going to make a bit of difference in your skewed perception of your physical self.

There are two main problems at work in body-image distortion: biochemical changes resulting from undereating that affect body-image perception, and an unrealistic standard of thinness that inspires undereating. Most of the first half of the book is about the initial problem, which is a function of adaptation, although exactly how body-image changes are involved is not clear. We've touched on the second problem in this chapter, mainly with some suggestions for loosening the thinness ideal of our culture. Remember that the unrealistic standard for thinness in our culture is the critical setup for eating problems. Without it we'd all be busier and happier concerning ourselves with other things.

Psycho-emotional pain is created by the discrepancy between reality (what is) and the ideal (what we want). This discrepancy creates a tension or discomfort—pain. The presumption is that the ideal is certainly good, right, desirable and even necessary to obtain, and conversely, that reality is bad, ugly, terrible and even intolerable.

The pain of having, or thinking we have, a too-heavy body is, for most eating-disturbed people, very painful if not intolerable. Accepting it isn't a possibility. We think we must change it, forcing our bodies toward the ideal size and shape, often against all good judgment, common sense and genetic programming. The grave pain we experience is the powerful motivating force behind our avoidance of food. In fact it is, for us, greater than the pain of starvation.

Our notion of the ideal body comes predominantly from our culture. Although some eating-disturbed individuals have a history of pressure to be thinner from their families, most do not. So most of us learn how our bodies should look from complete strangers—designers, photographers, advertising firms and models. The food jail door is locked by people we don't even know.

CHANGING REALITY VS. CHANGING YOUR THINKING

There are two ways to deal with the pain of not fitting the very thin cultural ideal for body shape. The first one is familiar: try to get smaller by the only known means available—undereating. And the second one may never have occurred to you: change your expectations, set your own personal standard. As we've discovered, the first way of coping is at the very heart of eating problems. And it really isn't a viable choice because it is a trap that makes people sick.

Can you pick more realistic expectations for yourself? Is it possible to defy the standard set by anonymous fashion gurus? Is there any way to ignore this pervasive cultural pressure to be thinner and live in peace with your imperfect body? Perhaps. And maybe not. It depends.

NEW EXPECTATIONS

The best way to adjust your own expectations for your body and lessen your body-image pain is to look realistically at your body standard and then at your eating and anti-eating history. Have you ever achieved your goal? At what price? Are you willing to continue to be at war with your body in an attempt to look a certain way? Are you willing to continue to jeopardize your health in order to try to be a certain weight? Would being diagnosed with a life-threatening illness change your priorities?

Facing some very hard facts can really open your eyes to the jail you're in and may begin to motivate you to consider breaking free someday. It's your relentless expectation to be ever thinner that puts you in jail, your belief that you must eat less that locks the jail door and the fear of letting go of your eating-control tactics that deadbolts you in.

RELATIVITY TRAINING— TAKING A LOOK AT YOUR GENES

Does your heredity point to extreme leanness as a possibility for you? Probably not. It doesn't for most of us. But some people do come from very lanky families, and they may be naturally very thin themselves. Many fashion models get started when their naturally tall and very thin frames attract model talent scouts. By normal medical standards, these women are often technically underweight or overtall, but they may be just right for their unique frames and body types. Their bodies are not in the majority, though. Although there are more of them during adolescence because lankiness is more common at that stage of development, natural superthins are rather uncommon by adulthood.

Are your parents tall and lean? Have they always been thin, naturally? Are your aunts and uncles on the lanky side, too? If you can say yes to all three questions then you may have a natural affinity for extra thinness. Although natural leanness is no immunization against eating disturbances, and may even predispose some to anorexia, your genetics can make staying thin a bit easier as your eating normalizes. Unfortunately, though, it has no benefit whatsoever for getting your distorted body image back into shape.

But what if you are like most people whose parents and close relatives are medium-framed and perhaps a bit plump in later adulthood? There are usually a few stocky people mixed into this family type. What's your prognosis for achieving and keeping The Very Thin Ideal with genes like this? Almost zero. Even if you are willing to sign up for self-starvation and disturbed eating for the rest of your life, it is unlikely that you'll get where you want to go without health-threatening anorexia. And the effort and damage is sure to cost you dearly.

And some of us come from families where one or both parents are actually overweight, or endlessly fighting the battle of the bulge with potions, powders, meetings and menus. These families usually come complete with a scattering of overweight aunts and uncles, cousins and siblings. It is easier to understand why people with families like these would develop crazy eating patterns than those from naturally thin families because overweight is all around, threatening and bringing pain. But all kinds of people develop eating troubles because all kinds of people want to be thinner and believe that simply eating less than they need will make them so.

What's the point of checking your family out when you're designing new expectations for your body shape? Your family's physical traits are your best reference point for making a reality check. This doesn't mean that you're doomed to being overweight if you come from a heavier family. It does mean that you need to factor in your family's genetics in order to have a realistic sense of your natural shape tendencies. Often, people with eating disorders are violating their health in a futile attempt to re-create their bodies' genetic blueprint.

Doris had been bulimic for six years. She identified her main motivation for self-starvation as "thin thighs." Her thighs disgusted her, she said, and made clothes-buying difficult. Her waist, like her upper body, was small. She would have worn a size seven if it hadn't been for her thick thighs and bottom. She had only managed to get them thin enough once in the years of her eating disorder, and that lasted only a few months.

Doris had never really looked at the price she was paying for this goal, which, when she took her family into consideration, was unattainable. One serious look at her parents and their families gave Doris a jolt of reality. She was obviously predestined to have disproportionate legs.

Once she accepted this fact and stopped starving herself, Doris began to look for some different ways to cope with her thick thighs. She consulted a wardrobe expert and found some practical new ways to flatter her shape with clothes. And by talking to a trainer, she discovered that some exercises she was doing were actually building the leg muscles that she wanted to tone down. Naturally, she changed those. And, ironically, Doris also faced the fact that all her dieting had left her upper body emaciated, which made her look even more out of proportion. That gave her added incentive to stay off the Cycle and start upper-body conditioning to build up her shoulders and arms. A body-image support group helped Doris keep her thighs in perspective, which she has done succesfully for the two years since conquering her eating disorder.

A LESSON IN PERSPECTIVE—TAKING A LOOK AT YOUR DIET HISTORY

Perhaps The Thin Ideal you've pursued for two, five or more years has been worthwhile to you. Maybe being thin or extremely thin is at the very core of your goals in life. Some say it is. But others are troubled and angered at the idea that being thin enough has controlled and even destroyed so much in their lives. They are disgusted with themselves for the high price they've paid to buy the thinness idol, and they are uncertain about how to live without it at the center of their identity. What about you?

1. How long have you been trying to get thinner by restricting your food intake?
2. How has The Thin Ideal affected your life? Make a list, including career, family, relationships, physical health, emotional health and education.
3. Have your efforts to achieve thinness been effective? For how long? At what price?
4. Have the benefits of your eating struggles been worthwhile in light of the price you've paid?
5. Do you believe that your eating disturbance will keep you thin indefinitely? At what cost?
6. Are you willing to continue your crazy eating habits in order to control your weight?
7. Are you able to continue your disturbed eating patterns to control your weight?
8. Do you feel capable of making a choice about your eating or are you trapped and paralyzed in food jail?

TAKING A LOOK AHEAD—YOUR DIET FUTURE

Picture yourself ten years from now. First, paint your eating problem and The Thin Ideal into the picture. This picture is likely to be somewhat like the look back at your diet history if your eating troubles are not severe. You are still struggling with hunger every day, still ritualizing what you eat, still popping laxatives to get rid of that bloated feeling, still angry and frustrated at your body, hating your shape and size, whatever they are. Going out to eat and parties are still threatening, compliments about your looks still suspect, depression and mood swings still common. And your weight hasn't changed much, unless it's gone up.

Seriously underweight anorectics and severe bulimics who purge chronically may not have to tolerate this unhappy picture ten years from now because they might be dead. If they do survive, their lives will still be locked in by The Thin Ideal and their chances of recovery very slim indeed. They may or may not reach that ideal, but their disorder will be obvious in their appearance, that's for sure.

Now look ten years down the road at a whole, emancipated person, free from disturbed eating. The Thin Ideal is a vague memory, like grade school. You outgrew it; you graduated. Your perspective got bigger and you learned to take care of your body for the sake of health and energy and life. The thin god was dethroned, you were set free. What is your life like now?

You are well and active. No one would ever suspect that you had trouble with your eating at one time. You eat plenty of good food. You don't think about eating much because you are so busy doing things you like and other things you must do. Your life revolves around your family, friends, work and interests. You can remember the time when it didn't, it couldn't, but it's like remembering a bad dream.

What'll it be? You hold the rudder to this boat, you set the sail.

O.P.I.O.O.M. ADDICTION

O.P.I.O.O.M. stands for Other People's Inferred Opinions of Me. Most people with eating disorders with whom I've worked are inordinately preoccupied with how others view their bodies, and I was, too, when I was afflicted. They seem to tune into other people's standards for their bodies, as if they didn't have enough body-image problems of their own! The "Inferred" is important because it points to the fact that these opinions are actually unknown, perhaps nonexistent, and always thought to be at least as critical and rejecting as their own. People with eating disturbances think they can figure out what others are thinking about their bodies, and so infer these alleged opinions. But for each sick one who plays, this is a game of solitaire, and a miserable one.

As if it weren't enough to have a stranglehold on yourself because of the goddess Thin—oh, no, eating disturbances are not such kind or moderate taskmasters—other "you're not thin enough" monsters must be brought in from outside, even imaginary ones. We care about others' opinions because that is a part of being socialized. It's not wrong and it's not necessarily destructive, excepting those times when this concern gets extreme. What to do?

Whenever I complained about what everybody else might think, my mother would remind me coolly, "Don't worry about what others are thinking about you because they're not thinking about you at all." It's a real blow to that narcissistic streak in all of us. And it's true. We're busy thinking about our own problems and our own bodies and our own lives. We'd like to be the center of the universe, I guess, but we're not. No, not you either.

Here's an exercise for finding your little place in the big scheme of things:

Think of yourself in your house with all the rooms and furniture, and other people who live there if you don't live alone.

Then imagine yourself in your neighborhood, and all the houses and streets and trees and cars and kids and basketball hoops.

Now back up a bit to see yourself in your entire city, with all the neighborhoods strung together, with stores and streetlights, boulevards and parks.

Now go another step into space, and see yourself in your whole country, one person among millions and millions of others.

Last, try to picture yourself as a teeny part of the whole planet, and then into outer space, as part of our whole galaxy.

Hold that last perspective. How thin are you now? Who cares?

CHAPTER 7

Breakout: How Eight Courageous Women Escaped from Food Jail

THE IDEA OF HAVING A HEALTHFUL WAY OF EATING, AN acceptable body image and a balanced life may seem like a pipe dream to some of you reading this book. It usually does to anyone stuck in food jail. The dream of having a healthy body and relationship with food seems so impossible from behind the bars of an eating disorder that most need evidence that it is possible. My clients often ask me for stories, examples of others who have gotten well. They ask questions about these success stories, such as "How long did it take?" "Did she gain weight?" "How much?" "How long before she was OK with her body?" "Any relapses?"

In this chapter are just a few of the dozens of stories I have been told about or witnessed, to help you understand what real people cope with in their quest for freedom from eating problems. These stories offer you evidence that true recovery is possible, and a glimpse of life after eating disturbances from the perspective of the individuals who have escaped from the food jail.

• "I HAD TO DO THIS OR DIE"—*Candy D.*

A business owner, wife and mother of a two-year-old daughter, Candy D. recalls her long and dangerous road to food jail with a shiver of fear and then relief.

Candy's quest for thinness began very early, as it often does for anorectics. When she was just nine years old Candy's ten- and eleven-year-old friends were dieters, and she joined their anti-eating lifestyle in order to be accepted, she says. Actually, Candy had already been introduced to her alleged weight problem and diet tactics at home, so she was primed for the peer influence that followed. Although Candy was a good athlete and student, she doesn't remember being acknowledged much for these qualities. She hoped to find in dieting and getting thinner the attention she was missing.

Most very young dieters are extreme in their attempts to lose weight and Candy was no exception. She literally starved herself for as long as she could take it, which was a few days to a week at most. Then she'd overeat for a day or two when she couldn't seem to control her eating. She lost weight and she gained it back in this pattern. Gradually, during her teens, she gained more than she lost.

After about ten years of up-and-down dieting, Candy's weight had crept up to 175 and felt very uncomfortable to her, even though her five-foot nine-inch large-boned frame carried it well. At nineteen she decided not to go on a diet, since the weight loss never lasted. Inspired by a popular spiritual approach to weight control, Candy simply limited her portions, eating only small amounts of food throughout the day. Her hunger level was so intense, she was so famished and tempted to binge, that she actually prayed for God's help to get through a dinner out or a party. But since she wasn't very physically active, Candy's extreme food restriction seemed reasonable to her.

Candy lost weight. In fact, she was down to 140 in just a few months. She felt better, except for the nagging hunger she had to live with. And she looked quite thin at that weight, but she thought she should drop another ten or fifteen pounds just for insurance against her tendency to rebound. So she kept up the same routine, eating very small amounts of food almost devoid of fat when she absolutely had to eat.

Candy's weight continued to drop. When it got down to 115 pounds her husband told her to stop dieting. Her parents became concerned and asked her to see a doctor for a checkup. But Candy felt pretty good. She was finally far enough away from the overweight cliff that she felt secure about not gaining the weight back. Clothes hung on her. People at work noticed and made comments about her diet, and asked her questions with obvious envy. Candy enjoyed the attention. She felt special because of her thinness. She wasn't going to give it up.

The now tiny nonfat meals Candy had adopted as a means to her new very thin shape continued. She assumed that her weight would level off on its own, and she felt afraid to change her routine at this point. Deep down Candy knew she was thin—too thin really—but she couldn't take the chance of gaining back the weight she'd lost. She never wanted to go back to being heavy because she was just like everyone else when she was overweight.

Candy's eating had gradually become more and more rigid. She discovered that she was locked into an eating pattern that she couldn't break away from, and it began to frighten her. She did a lot of rationalizing about this to manage her fear. Lots of people eat this way, most models are as thin as I am, there is nothing wrong with controlling your eating—it's healthy and it shows self-discipline, she told herself.

Her inflexible and minimal eating rituals brought still more weight loss. At 106 pounds Candy began to have occasional chest pains, and for the first time in her weight-control efforts she was really alarmed—afraid for her health and even afraid for her life.

For four years Candy's weight hovered around 105 pounds. Her husband and parents shared her fear, although Candy didn't tell them everything. She didn't want to alarm them. Besides the chest pain, she was frequently dizzy, and had headaches, weakness and many fainting spells. She couldn't sleep much anymore and her hair was thin and dull. Her periods had stopped when her weight fell below 120 pounds.

Candy knew she was too thin. She even wanted to gain some weight—a little weight—but she couldn't. She was trapped by her fear of gaining too much weight. This fear provoked in her an intense need to maintain strict control of her eating. She knew she should eat more, but she was powerless to do it. She was locked in food jail.

Candy read a newspaper article about adaptation and the Naturally Thin Program. Although she didn't see herself as anorectic, she knew something was wrong with her eating patterns and she was sure this was her only chance to get well.

Candy had never been in treatment for anorexia, mainly because she never admitted that she had this disorder. Concerned as they were, no one in her family ever forced her into treatment. The only professional in her life who focused on her weight as a problem was her chiropractor, but even she never used the word "anorexia." So the traditional treatments for Candy's condition were never considered. It didn't matter now. All Candy knew was that the Naturally Thin ideas made sense and gave her the courage to start changing her eating.

Unsure of exactly what she was attempting to accomplish, Candy told her husband she was going to try it. He was thrilled because she'd been completely resistant to any changes in her eating until then. He was, along with Candy's whole family, very concerned about her health. And he wanted to have children—a dream that wouldn't be possible unless she got well, and soon. He knew instinctively that Candy could die from starvation if she didn't get help.

A very motivated student, Candy absorbed the Naturally Thin Program for breaking out of food jail quickly. This created some relief and hope in her as she gained weight, but it also brought fear. Candy was afraid to give the controls for her eating to her body. She now realized that she'd been in a severe famine for four years, so she knew she'd gain weight if she let go, but she didn't know how much or for how long. And the idea of losing her "thin identity" was very difficult. But it was not as fearful as the alternative—losing her life. Candy was convinced that she would die if she didn't do something about her weight and eating problems.

"I had to do this or die," Candy now admits matter-of-factly, but the path to normal eating and a healthy weight was harder and longer than she had imagined.

"Keep food with you, eat when you are hungry until you are full, never go hungry, eat only high-quality Real Food, drink plenty of water, never go hungry, don't undereat—ever, take food with you." The Naturally Thin principles echoed in Candy's head day and night as she tried to apply them. She very gradually increased her portions, and as she did she discovered that she obsessed less about food. Then she worked on breaking down her rigid controls by eating "forbidden foods" occasionally, and eating at "forbidden times," like between meals, and in "forbidden places," like her car or office.

As she made adjustments, Candy needed a lot of support, especially at certain crisis times. She regularly experienced anxiety attacks and "freaked out" about her new eating behavior, fearful of gaining huge amounts of weight overnight. And when she did notice that she was actually gaining weight, she was often overwhelmed with panic and tempted to try to regain control of her eating. These temptations were usually short-lived, though, because she knew by the time she was a few weeks into it that she could never go back to anorectic eating. It wasn't physically possible for her once she had really given the controls to her body. So

there was only one way left for her to go—forward. She had eaten
herself into a narrow passageway, one leading to her liberation.

Candy got most of her support from her husband, and from her
family as well. She didn't tell anyone at her job about what she
was doing because she was afraid they wouldn't understand, and
she felt embarrassed about her eating disorder. Her family was
completely supportive, she says, because they knew if she didn't
change she wouldn't make it. One Christmas her dad had told
Candy he knew it was her last unless she got some help. Like
most families of anorectics, Candy's had faced that reality a long
time before she did.

Candy needed much reassurance as she let go of her own rules
and gave her body more and more power to control her eating.
Her husband told her over and over again, "You're doing the right
thing, I'm so proud of you for doing it, I love you." This is what I
call "personal support." He didn't try to counsel Candy or give her
advice. He just reminded her of some basic realities that she
needed to hear. His role wasn't complicated but he was invaluable, boosting her confidence and security every day, especially
while she was overweight.

Candy asked me for a different sort of support, "counselor support." Usually in a panic, she would contact me for advice, direction, specific reassurance and, occasionally, prophecy.

Here's a typical conversation:

CANDY: Hello, Jean?

JEAN: Yes?

CANDY: Oh, thank God! I just have to talk to you! I'm scared,
Jean. I mean, really scared.

JEAN: What's going on?

CANDY: I'm so hungry! I'm just ravenous! And I'm scared that
this gigantic hunger is going to make me huge again.

JEAN: Candy, you never were huge. But you're afraid your
hunger, if you keep eating, will lead you back to being overweight?

CANDY: I am eating—all the time, and I'm gaining. I started out eating a little more, but now I'm eating a lot more, and I don't think I can stop it anymore. My body is definitely in control. I don't know how much weight I've gained because you said to stay off the scale. But my clothes are tight—all of them. I know you said I'd gain, but it's one thing to talk about it and another to actually see the weight on your body.

JEAN: I need to see what you mean by eating all the time. What exactly did you eat yesterday?

CANDY: I got up at six and immediately had a banana and a big bowl of cornflakes with skim milk, and two pieces of toast with jelly. Then at eight-fifteen I was hungry and had an English muffin and a big glob of low-fat cottage cheese with orange juice—a big glass. At eleven I ate a tuna salad sandwich, coleslaw and a mineral water plus a few bites of leftover spaghetti. When I got hungry at about two I had a peanut butter and olive sandwich and a bunch of carrot sticks dipped in ranch dressing. Then I ate the rest of the leftover spaghetti—a huge plate—and two apples at around four-forty-five. I couldn't eat supper with my husband at six because I was too full, but I got hungry again at seven-thirty and had a toasted bagel with jelly and a huge salad. Skim milk just before bed.

JEAN: Excellent. I think you're eating enough. You're never, ever going hungry?

CANDY: What do you think? No!

JEAN: Candy, do you remember why you are eating so much and gaining weight?

CANDY (pause): Because I need to. Because I've been in a famine and my body has to compensate for that before it can level off at a healthier weight.

JEAN: Right. And how far up is your weight going to go?

CANDY: As far as it needs to, to protect me from any future famines.

JEAN: And will there be any future famines for your body, Candy?

CANDY: Not if I can help it! No, there won't be any more famines for my body.

JEAN: That's right, the famines are over. But your body doesn't know it yet. Your job is to convince it that the famines are over forever. You'll never go hungry again. Candy, are you taking food with you so you never get stranded without something to eat?

CANDY: Absolutely. I always have food with me, and I'll eat it anywhere, anytime I get hungry. I don't care what anybody thinks—and some people think I'm nuts!

JEAN: And how's your preoccupation with food?

CANDY: You know, that's the part that really shocks me. Sometimes I go for an hour or even two when I'm not hungry, and I don't even think about food or eating at all. You said this would happen, but I didn't believe you. I've been so obsessed with food for so long . . .

JEAN: That's a good sign. And your relentless hunger signals are a good sign, too.

CANDY: Really? I thought they were a disaster in the making.

JEAN: No, they're a good sign because they mean that your body is getting the message you're trying to send—that the famines are over. Your increased hunger means your body is responding to the change in the food supply in a healthy way. It's a big piece in the get-well plan for you.

CANDY: That's good to know. I feel better, but what do I do about my clothes? Tight clothes send me into a total panic.

JEAN: Definitely get bigger clothes, at Goodwill, consignment shops, bigger friends, wherever. This is important to keep your anxiety manageable. Dress comfortably. If something doesn't fit, the clothes are wrong, not your body.

CANDY: I'll try to remember that. This is really hard—harder than I thought. Do you still think I can do it?

JEAN: You are doing it. You're doing great. Keep going.

CANDY: OK. But I'm still scared.

Candy gained weight very gradually for about a year on the Naturally Thin Program. She knew she'd overshoot her ideal weight because of the severity of the famine she'd been on, but knowing that didn't make it any easier for her when it happened. Once a co-worker actually asked her when her baby was due, and she wasn't pregnant! But by the time that happened, Candy was in a pretty good place with her body. It shook her up a little anyway.

A clear sign of progress came when Candy's periods started again after just a few months of eating freely. This boost was counterbalanced by the loss of her "thin identity." It was tough for Candy to give up the physical trait that she thought made her unique, but the freedom she gained in her eating and in her life made it more tolerable.

After the initial gain Candy leveled off. Just when she was feeling relieved, she gained a bit more. Finally she plateaued for about ten months, and then gradually started losing weight, eating freely the whole time. She had dropped about twenty pounds when she was jolted by frightening news: she really was pregnant. This was an accident. She called me in near hysterics, afraid she'd gain fifty or more pounds during the pregnancy.

She didn't. Candy did not gain any weight at all the first six months of her pregnancy. She was not restricting her eating at all, and in fact, she was eating a great deal of good food, and often (six or seven meals a day with fruit and granola bars between meals). Candy gained only fifteen pounds during her full-term pregnancy. She delivered a beautiful, healthy girl, and shortly afterward, started losing weight again, naturally. She complained to me during this time that she had to eat almost constantly to keep up with her appetite, especially for the first few months of breastfeeding. Her weight decreased methodically. It seemed the more she ate, the less she weighed. By ten months postpartum, Candy leveled off at about 145. Nice and thin for a woman five nine.

She called me: "Jean, I can't believe it! I'm thin! I mean, I'm really thin! And I'm still eating all the time. I'm naturally thin!"

Candy went through fire to break out of food jail—a period of significant overweight. The fear of it keeps many in jail indefinitely. The threat of death pushed her to face it. And she did. Candy tackled her fear squarely and courageously, coped with the loss and pain, and broke free into a new life—a life she never thought possible.

• "I THOUGHT OF SUICIDE ALMOST CONSTANTLY"—*Patty M.*

An elementary school teacher, wife and mother of four, Patty didn't remember ever not hating her body. Although she had always had a rather slight frame, she couldn't recall ever feeling thin enough or physically feminine. Growing up in a large family with lots of sisters who were dieting and obsessed with their weight, she possibly learned some of her body-image troubles from home. The way she ultimately chose to deal with them, however, was unique in her family.

An attractive and petite woman, Patty dieted off and on throughout high school. She tolerated the ups and downs of her weight pretty well, although she often felt depressed and unattractive during that time. Throughout college the dieting continued fairly successfully while Patty was extremely busy in theater productions. "It was like being on diet pills then, I was so keyed up—I couldn't eat most of the time," she recalls.

During her senior year in college Patty had just successfully lost weight by starving herself when she met the man she would later marry. An emotionally abusive traveling salesman, he added to Patty's deep insecurities about her body by making mean comments about her eating and body shape. Two years after the wedding, a post-famine pregnancy and the birth of her first baby brought Patty to a new low in her relationship with her body. Her husband, an extremely thin person, berated her for gaining weight during her pregnancy. His cruel remarks continued even when she was perfectly thin between babies. All this affected Patty's body image deeply, although she tried to ignore him. Ultimately they divorced, but much damage was done.

Reeling emotionally from the divorce and the responsibilities of now two small children, Patty developed multiple food allergies. It got to the point where she could eat only a few foods without reacting with sneezes, an itchy throat and a runny nose. This was probably related to the high stress level in her life. As a result of these sensitivities, plus her inordinate concern about her weight,

Patty became extremely rigid in her eating patterns, exerting strict control over every morsel of food that she allowed in her mouth. A typical lunch for her at this time consisted of steamed cabbage and bottled water.

Depression and thoughts of suicide closed in on Patty like a dark storm. The stress, fear, pain and anger were an unbearable load, and coupled with the frustration of the weight she had gained in her transition to independence, Patty knew something had to give. And it did. One night she lost control and began to eat everything in sight—chips, dips, cheese, ice cream—all the foods she knew she reacted to and caused her to bloat and gain weight. But Patty couldn't control the powerful urge within her. She saw herself from outside, as if she were another person, and she simply could not stop. She realized, even while she ate, that she would react to these foods with allergic symptoms and weight gain.

So Patty "undid" the binge by throwing up. It wasn't hard. In fact, it was a great relief. When she stood up from her position over the toilet and looked at herself in the bathroom mirror, she saw a tired, old woman with bloodshot eyes. She was twenty-eight.

At first she binged and purged only twice a week, but within a few months Patty was famine-feast-purge Cycling twice a day and sometimes more. Her famines, with rigid eating controls and food group restrictions, continued another six years, and the feasting binges and desperate purges continued exactly that long, too. She didn't know there was a pattern in her eating disorder, that there was a relationship between her food restriction and her overeating, her fear of getting fat and her purging. She thought it was stress that made her throw up. In fact, she was convinced, from reading articles about eating disorders and talking to a counselor, that her bulimia was about her repressed anger at her ex-husband and her parents.

When she learned about the FeaFam Cycle, Patty didn't believe it explained her whole tormented relationship with food. She was still convinced that her emotions played a major role in her eating struggle. In fact, she knew they did because she felt so upset or angry when she was throwing up. Besides, although the FeaFam Cycle made sense to her, Patty admits that it was very difficult to give up the feeling of control that counting calories, restricting food groups, etc., gave her. She wasn't ready to let go that much, at least not for a while.

Eventually, though, Patty found herself trying to eat more in spite of her skepticism. About the same time she stopped weighing herself, and stopped wearing tight clothes that pressured her to avoid eating. All these steps helped Patty to relax a bit, to get out from under the constant obsessing about food. "The first astounding change from my starting to eat more was that I stopped thinking of food every second of the day and night. That's when I began to see that bingeing would happen only after going hungry," she recalls.

Patty persevered in eating more and a greater variety of foods, and sometime during the next year, almost mysteriously, she stopped bingeing. Her last binge occurred about ten months after she began trying to eat more. And, of course, her last purging happened then, too. Instead of anger, Patty discovered that undereating was the real culprit behind her binges, and that her intense fear of weight gain had provoked her to purge.

That was seven years ago. Patty has since remarried and has had two more babies, gaining and losing weight without concern. ("The weight gain was the easiest part of those pregnancies!" she claims, as evidence of her newfound balance.) Her years of bulimia are like a thick fog in her memory, she says, part of a dark, sad time in her life. Patty is so far from troubled eating now that she says she cannot imagine how she ever lived the way she did, starving and bingeing and throwing up. It's as if she had been caught up in a nightmare during that time in her life and finally woke up to a whole new world.

This is how Patty sums up her transformation: "When I was on the Cycle my thoughts centered on food and my body almost all the time—nearly all my energy went into it. My main concern now is making sure I get enough food, period. The parts of eating that I have to work on are getting plenty of fruits and veggies and water every day. Pretty normal concerns I'd say. I have not gotten on a scale since 1984 (except for prenatal care). I know my weight is stable because my clothes fit the same. And I refuse to wear clothes that are tight. I guess I feel a tremendous freedom that I never felt all those years of dieting and bingeing."

• "I WOULD GO TO THE GROCERY STORE IN THE MIDDLE OF THE NIGHT—IN MY PAJAMAS!"—*Connie I.*

A single business manager/consultant, Connie told me that her eating disorder history just wasn't that interesting. But I found that it was "interesting" enough to get her into big eating trouble. She had once called the food jail she was in "compulsive eating."

Connie "discovered" that she was overweight when she was a freshman in high school. A senior boy watching her swimming practice impulsively called her plump and she took it to heart. Connie's relationship with her body wasn't normal again for years. Dieting became her way of life.

The first dozen or so diet plans Connie tried were faddish, extreme and probably dangerous. She lost weight on every one, for a while. Connie tolerated the terrible hunger she experienced on these diets and developed coping skills to stay with the various plans. For example, she learned to exercise when she got hungry, instead of eating, and drank gallons of diet pop, coffee and tea, which were usually allowed. She kept her refrigerator devoid of anything that wasn't on her diet. She never ate out, and if she had to eat at a friend's she took her own food.

Usually between three and nine months after these early diets began, Connie would lose her grip on her appetite. She experienced powerful, sometimes overwhelming cravings for sweets, especially. One of her favorite binge foods was Twinkies. She never kept them on hand because she knew she'd eat them if she did. But when her hunger was on the rampage, Connie found a way to get the foods she craved.

"At night I seemed more vulnerable to my compulsive eating," she recalls. "I was absolutely at the mercy of my cravings, especially after about eleven o'clock. I'd try to go to bed to keep myself from bingeing, but that didn't usually stop me. I would actually get out of bed and go to the grocery store, for Twinkies and cookies and donuts and ice cream, in my pajamas, in the middle of the night. Of course, I wore a trench coat over my PJs, but one time, as I was pondering my choice of delicacies, the thought occurred to me, I don't have any underwear on. I'm grocery shopping in a nightie without underwear. I must be sick."

Overeaters Anonymous was supposed to help people like Connie, so she went to a few meetings. She pledged abstinence from white flour, sugar and all food between meals. Of course she limited her overall intake of food at mealtimes as well because she was twenty-five pounds overweight. This abstinence plan eliminated all her binge foods and her opportunity to eat at the time she usually binged. It was a great plan. She got support and felt understood at OA. She stuck with it for five weeks.

As Connie continued her dieting efforts, she noticed that losing

weight became more difficult for her, and her rebound weight
gain was faster. And she couldn't stay with a diet for more than a
few weeks anymore. The cravings and nighttime binges came
much sooner after she started a new weight-loss program. In fact,
she found herself struggling with cravings most of the time now.
These two facts were immensely discouraging to Connie, who finally gave up on her body. She had learned at OA that she was
hopelessly addicted to food, and she couldn't get her addiction
under control, even with the help of her Higher Power. Connie
was under lock and key in food jail.

"Will I really stop bingeing? I won't eat and eat and eat and
never stop? I won't weigh three hundred pounds in six months?"
Connie worried. She was understandably anxious about eating
more—she felt as though she were already eating far too much!
Her appetite had been so extreme for so long and was completely
uncontrollable about half the time now. The idea of letting her
body manage her food intake almost sent her into hysterics. But
she understood the Feast or Famine Cycle and passionately hoped
it really did apply to her. At any rate, she decided there was no
other way for her to go.

The first few months getting off the Cycle were very stressful
for Connie. Her anxiety level was constantly high and her confidence low. Her first glimmer of hope came about seven weeks
into her new eating-by-demand routine when she abruptly
stopped eating halfway through a delicious seafood dinner. She
absolutely could not continue eating. She was so startled that at
first she thought she must be sick. Then she realized that this was
supposed to happen when her body finally got enough food over
a long enough time to lower her appetite. Connie was overwhelmed, and so relieved that she burst into tears, right there in
the restaurant.

"I made a total fool of myself," she remembers. "I think the
waiter thought someone had died. I just couldn't contain the relief
I felt—that my body could control my eating and actually stop me
from eating more. The whole key for me was eating enough—
something I never would have figured out in a million years."

Connie eventually plateaued at a higher weight than she had
hoped for, but she says she doesn't really care. "The weight is
nothing compared to the crazy way I was living," she explains. "I
still weigh less than I did most of the time I was on the Cycle, and
now I can live and eat like a normal human being—I'm free."

• "I KNEW ABOUT THIS PATH FOR FOUR YEARS BEFORE I COULD TAKE IT"—*Marta M.*

One of those chubby, frumpy kids who grew into a beauty, Marta learned very early that being thin was important. Her younger sister was chosen as a child model when Marta was just nine and too fat to try out. Although it impressed her that her life could be so affected by her weight, Marta didn't do anything about it until she was fifteen, when she started dieting and lost twenty pounds. She also got contact lenses, bleached her hair blond and learned how to use makeup. Even her parents were startled, Marta was so transformed.

Chosen to model for a local modeling agency when she was seventeen, Marta basked in the limelight. She was a favorite of Nan, the owner of the agency, who encouraged her to pursue modeling as a career. Marta looked up to Nan and hung on her every word, flattered by her special interest in her. So when Nan suggested that Marta would improve her chances of success by losing ten pounds, Marta set out to do it, though she was already very thin.

Before Nan's comment Marta's diet was quite restrictive—vegetarian, very low fat, strictly three meals a day. Where could she cut back? Skip lunch. Drink water instead. Exercise more. Increase workouts to six days a week instead of three. She could do this. It worked for her when she was fifteen and she could do it now at nineteen.

And she did. Her weight dropped more than ten pounds. One of the other models introduced her to diuretics, which helped with bloating, especially during the two weeks before her period. Clothes literally hung on her, and Nan said that's what the big agencies wanted—superthin. Nan sent Marta to L.A. to interview and test-shoot with one of the biggest agencies, and she was offered a job. She was ecstatic. This was big time, big money, big magazines, big fame. She didn't know it was big trouble, too.

Her first week, Marta was bowled over by the pace of her new job—half the days she literally worked over fourteen hours straight. Sometimes she'd actually be in front of a camera for more than three hours at a time—a grueling stretch to be posing. She nearly fainted every day at least once. She felt dizzy and couldn't concentrate at times. One of the agency staff could see that something was wrong and told Marta to see the agency's doctor.

When the doctor pulled her gown apart to listen to her lungs he knew what the problem was. Marta's bones protruded like those of women in lands struck by famine. The doctor told Marta she had to gain weight or she'd suffer permanent damage to her organs. He referred her to the eating disorders clinic in the area where he had referred many others before Marta, most in better health than she. Marta was so frightened by his comments that she went, "knowing" she couldn't gain much weight without jeopardizing her job, but maybe she could find out how to gain just enough to feel better and get rid of the dizziness.

The counselor encouraged Marta by pointing out the emotional components in anorexia. She suggested that Marta see a therapist and gave her a basic diet plan to follow. What a relief! This is emotional. I can handle that, Marta thought. She glanced at the daily diet sheet. It was more food than she ate in a week. This would never do. She'd gain too much weight and lose her job. I'll get more sleep, she promised herself.

The following week, after four days of rest, Marta felt better. In fact, she felt better than she had in a long time. She hadn't brought her special food supply with her one day, and feeling a bit cocky, she sat with the crew at a tableful of agency food. Marta normally never ate anything except her own food, but she was in such a mood this day, and the doctor had said she should gain some weight, that she made an exception and had a little salad with a cracker. Then she had a cookie—just one—and then she went into a kind of blackout. Although she was conscious, Marta says she was powerless to stop eating—like a robot under someone else's remote control. She ended up eating much more than she had planned, although it wasn't really more than a large meal. But to Marta, this was a gigantic binge, she was so unused to normal portions of anything, including water. She ate until it hurt and then she ate some more. She could not stop. When she finally pulled herself away, she instinctively raced for the bathroom—a portable toilet—and felt the food coming up into her mouth before she got the door open. "It felt as if I was losing all of my insides," she recalls.

This scene occurred only one other time while Marta modeled professionally. Most of the time she was able to maintain rigid eating rules that kept her extremely thin—emaciated, really. During this time she was able to keep her weight far below normal for the sake of her modeling career, but her health and her appearance continued to deteriorate. Finally, she lost her job.

Back home six months later, Marta learned about the Naturally Thin Program from an old friend. She was seeing a therapist at the time, working on the emotional conflicts that supposedly made her unwilling to eat enough, but she thought this physical approach was interesting, too. She even agreed with the adaptation idea and the various Cycles of eating disorders. She could see them in her crazy relationship with food, but she couldn't let go of her eating controls because she was just too afraid. The main emotional problem Marta could see clearly was her fear of gaining weight. She felt trapped, and she was.

Marta's anorexia gradually was displaced by bulimarexia—a common shift. The binge/purge cycles became more regular as the supercontrol she had once had over her eating waned. She began to binge more often and felt she had to vomit at those times to keep from gaining weight. Fortunately, Marta did gain some much-needed weight with this addition of regular bingeing, but her health and energy level were pitifully poor. She was only able to keep a sedentary part-time job as a receptionist, although she did find the strength to test for a modeling job or audition for a commercial acting job now and then. "I was never hired because I looked so sick," she now admits.

Four years after Marta's introduction to the Naturally Thin concepts, she decided to try to apply some of the ideas—the ones she could think about without having an anxiety attack. Firmly locked into the FeaFam Cycle, she was not convinced of this new approach's merit for her, but she was desperate to be released from her eating disorder lifestyle, which still revolved around food and weight, and kept her feeling chronically ill. Marta had never experienced any lasting changes in her eating from going to therapy and eating disorders programs, so she felt this was her only hope. Even that scared her. If this failed, what could she do?

Breaking the Cycle wasn't an all-or-nothing thing for Marta. There were stops and starts for months as she experimented with her appetite and changing eating behaviors. Consequently, it took a little over a year on and off the program for her binge/purge experiences to stop. She gained more weight during this time, but the Cycle was finally broken and she was so relieved to have a normal eating pattern, she didn't especially care. The door to complete eating freedom had opened and Marta walked through in a total time of less than three years—a full year less than the time it took her to decide to try breaking out of food jail.

Marta dropped the extra weight she had gained over the second and third years of Naturally Thin eating, as she kept carefully in touch with her hunger signals and stuck with high-quality foods. When her weight leveled off, she was surprised at how much she weighed, because she fit into clothes that she had worn fifteen pounds lighter. "That was just lucky," she confided to me, "because if they hadn't fit me I would have given them away. It doesn't really matter what my size is anymore. My body is finally happy.

"I don't know why it took me so long to do this," she continued. "I guess my eating problems didn't seem so bad for quite a while, as long as I could stay thin. I had to get ready, you know, be sick enough of being so sick to really want to get well, no excuses. Some people wake up more slowly than others. But for me, it was almost like coming back from the dead. It was so great to just have energy and not feel cold. I was never crazy about my periods, but I guess that's part of being healthy. The main thing is, I don't have to think about food all the time anymore. I just stick to eating good food and I never go hungry. In fact, I can't go hungry! Pretty simple plan, but it's a miracle for me."

• "I STUFFED M&Ms DOWN MY THROAT FASTER THAN I COULD SWALLOW THEM"—*Liz B.*

A loan officer, wife and mother of two young adults, Liz had been dubbed "butterball" when she was just twelve years old. She was chubby then, no doubt about it, but had never really noticed until a friend's dad put the label on her. This comment set Liz up for the many decisions she made that ultimately affected over three decades of her life. The friend's dad wasn't to blame—it was probably just a casual remark. The diet culture in America is responsible for the seduction that followed.

Liz knew about dieting from her mother, who was always on one diet program or another. Her mother was a little overweight, but talked about dieting a great deal. When Liz checked the "butterball" label out in a mirror she knew what she had to do, and her mother was eager to help. Together they joined TOPS (Take Off Pounds Sensibly). When she lost ten pounds, she was rewarded with a plaque and a big applause. But when she gained the weight back, she was given the "Piggy Award," a most embarrassing experience. She vowed never to go back, but she did, years later.

At nineteen Liz knew she needed more than a support group to lose weight, so she went to a doctor and got diet pills, or amphetamines. These little tablets were like a gift from heaven, Liz thought. They made losing weight (and cleaning her apartment) a breeze. These stimulant/appetite suppressants are known now as speed and are illegal. Liz knows why. She lost twenty-five pounds and stayed extremely thin as long as she was on the pills, about five years. But after she got married she decided to go off them because of her emotional reactivity and heart palpitations. In just one year Liz gained fifty pounds. The slender bride had disappeared in a hurry.

When the horror of her weight gain struck, amphetamines were no longer available, so Liz's only recourse was dieting. And diet she did. Every diet plan you can think of she tried, and several repeatedly. And Liz was a very successful dieter, winning awards from most of the groups she joined. The diet was the easy part for her. Maintenance was impossible. Just as soon as she reached her goal, or shortly thereafter, she began to eat—uncontrollably. Forty- or fifty-pound weight fluctuations went on for over thirty years.

Food binges had been a part of Liz's life for so long that she considered them normal. She was not alone. All her dieting friends (and that was all her friends) complained of the same struggle with their appetites. In fact, it was something that bonded them together, gave them something to talk about. Liz's compulsive eating was upsetting but never confusing to her. She knew what it was about—her body's defective appetite, her poor willpower, her sick lust for food. The first time the thought struck Liz that something might be seriously wrong with her was the day she reached her goal with Weight Watchers.

Liz ate nothing for two days before the weigh-in at her regular Weight Watchers meeting. She drank gallons of tea and diet pop to stave off the hunger and lose water weight. This wasn't all that difficult for Liz—she was in shape to go hungry, especially before meetings, in order to "make weight." She had only one pound to lose that last week, but it was coming off more slowly and her appetite was growing by leaps and bounds. She was determined. Weak and dehydrated, Liz weighed in and made her goal weight. She was relieved. Everyone applauded. She blushed and accepted her award. Others looked at her with envy thinking, If she can do it, I can do it!

From the meeting Liz drove straight to the drugstore to buy

M&Ms. She just wanted to reward herself. Waiting until she was safely inside her own home, Liz broke the bag open and began to shovel candies into her salivating mouth. Her hands were shaking and the M&Ms spilled onto the floor, bouncing and rolling all over. Hardly noticing, Liz made her way over to the sink, stuffing the morsels into her mouth like a drug-crazed addict. She wasn't swallowing them as fast as she was pushing them into her mouth, and she was forced to take a sip of water to keep from choking.

When Liz had pushed the whole two-pound bagful in, she finally looked up and out her window. There she saw her own reflection. At first she didn't recognize herself. The old, frightened, haggard woman she saw, with bulging cheeks and trembling hands, was someone else. She spit the chocolate left in her mouth into the sink and looked up again. "You have an eating disorder," she told the reflection out loud. Then she looked down and ate the candies she had spit out a moment before.

Overeaters Anonymous was filled with people, especially women, who did the things Liz did. They talked about their powerlessness over food, their addiction to it and the importance of following the program. They didn't talk about weight loss, which was a relief to Liz, who was rapidly gaining back the thirty pounds she'd lost with Weight Watchers this last time. By the time Liz's weight had peaked out again, she'd gained forty pounds and felt she absolutely needed a program for weight loss.

Overeaters Victorious is patterned after OA but includes a focus on weight loss as part of the program. With more emphasis on the "spiritual side of eating problems," OV taught Liz that her overeating was sinful and that she needed forgiveness and guidance from God to overcome it. OK, Liz thought, this is an approach I haven't tried. Maybe this is why my dieting always fails, why my eating is getting so bizarre. But spiritualizing her eating disturbance wasn't the answer for Liz either, and the binges continued to follow her attempts to lose weight.

Several diets, followed by severe eating bouts, later, Liz heard about the Naturally Thin Program for breaking out of food jail. She was excited by the idea of never having to diet again, but the notion of losing weight without dieting was beyond her. The possibility that her cravings and compulsive eating could be stopped—by eating—intrigued Liz. She was so desperate, so tired of the yo-yo diet cycle, so anxious to make peace with food, that Liz jumped wholeheartedly into the Naturally Thin Program.

"I'd gained back so much weight after diets that I didn't care about gaining at first. I just figured I would gain anyway, so why not enjoy it this one time?" Liz offers as an explanation for her fearlessness.

There was no hesitation for Liz, once she had made the decision to learn to eat. Her last binge happened about a week after she started—a half pan of brownies. It never happened again, ever. Liz just never overate from that time on, nor was she tempted. Her taste for sweets was gone by her fourth week of eating, something she had hoped for because it seemed to be the crux of her compulsive binges.

Liz's appetite changed so dramatically that, around her first anniversary of body-controlled eating, she was so disinterested in sweets that the three cakes that were brought to celebrate her birthday on separate occasions had no appeal for her and she turned all three down, much to the shock of her friends and family. This resistance was not about willpower, holiness, emotional health or abstinence. It was about eating enough, and she was, finally.

When Liz's husband, Herb, saw the transformation in her eating, and the changes in her whole attitude toward food and her body, he had to find out what she was up to. He had witnessed her weight fluctuations and her weird eating patterns for years. And although Liz had tried to hide her compulsive bingeing, Herb knew something was up when whole cakes disappeared while he was out of the house on a short errand. Herb was already convinced that whatever Liz was doing, it was definitely different. When he found out, he decided to join his wife and get his own eating straightened out. His eating troubles weren't nearly as dramatic as Liz's, but he was on the Feast or Famine Cycle and needed to kick his taste for fatty foods. And right along with Liz, he did.

Although it took about three years for Liz's weight to stabilize at a healthy place, she says her real recovery—getting a normal relationship with food—happened in only a few months of eating enough. "We're all trying to do it backwards—lose weight by having a sick relationship with food—and it never works," she explains. "You have to get right with food first, and the weight trouble gradually takes care of itself. You just can't believe it until it happens to you, and then it's like getting your whole life back."

• "THIS PROGRAM RUINED ME AS AN EMOTIONAL BINGER"—
Sally P.

Describing her upbringing in "dietland," Sally says she does not remember a time when she wasn't conscious of her weight and her eating. Although her photos as a child and early adolescent show no signs of excess weight, Sally felt she was fat from the time she was five. These inconsistencies reflect the sad fact that a distorted body image is all it takes to get young girls caught up in dieting. Her father was no help, nicknaming her Chub when she was about seven years old.

A day-care provider and single mother of three small boys, Sally winces as she looks back on her years growing up. "My mother's whole life was dieting," Sally remembers. "She didn't exactly tell me I was fat, but I definitely got the message that I would be if I didn't diet. By the time I was ten years old, I was in a 'diet club' with two other girls my age."

Sally was thirteen years old when she experienced what she recognized as her first emotionally induced binge. An older boy she had been infatuated with jilted her, and the pain of rejection and loss sent her into a two-day sweets orgy. Of course, she'd been dieting strenuously in order to impress this particular guy, but she never associated the binge with her dieting. All she saw was the fifty pounds she would probably gain if she didn't regain control, so she doubled her dieting efforts after that.

Then it happened again when Sally failed an important algebra test. And again when her sister got married. And once more after a friend moved out of town. And again when a very attractive date stood her up. And again when . . . And again when . . . Every time the trigger for bingeing was some painful emotion. Sally began to see herself as emotionally crippled—a compulsive emotional overeater.

Gradually, the binges outweighed Sally's success at dieting and she gained weight. The extra weight was obvious to others, but this never-ending fight between Sally and her body was a secret. Sally was so ashamed of her bizarre episodes of gorging on donuts and cookies and brownies and fudge and ice cream and peanut butter that she took care to hide evidence of the battle from everyone. Who would understand? she thought. When she married at twenty, even her husband knew nothing of her crazy eating patterns.

Eight years of a rocky marriage and three babies later, the patterns were still going strong. Sally had resigned herself to it: When she got upset she binged. It had been that way for so long that sometimes it seemed normal to her, although she knew people who didn't binge just because they had problems. Deep down Sally felt defective—that there was something terribly wrong with her, and there was. She just didn't have a clue as to what it was. Her husband actually contributed to the seriousness of her problem by berating her for being overweight. His jabs and cruel remarks helped keep the pressure on her to diet, which, of course, she did.

Sally joined a co-dependence support group and learned about the Feast or Famine Cycle from a group member. "It made sense to me instantly. My whole life was geared to staying away from food, and when pain or stress came along, my willpower broke down under the load. I finally saw why I binged when I got upset. I needed to binge. I was starving. I was dying for food." Sally was ready to change. Although she had given up hope of getting thin permanently, she just wanted to get off this battlefield with her body and eat like regular people.

Giving up calorie counting, fat gram counting and portion control wasn't easy for Sally because these control tactics had become as obsessive as her preoccupation with food. Learning to tune in to hunger signals, eat on time, avoid the scale and stop buying "diet foods" were challenging, too: "It seemed as if my whole life was turned upside down," she explains. "Everything I had been doing with food my entire life had to be undone, and I had to learn to do almost the exact opposite. It made me feel crazy for a while." Sally persevered anyway, she says, because she believed the Naturally Thin principles. "Besides," she adds, "I really was crazy when I was starving and bingeing. Feeling a bit nuts on the way to normal didn't seem like too high a price to pay to get my body and my head straightened out."

The ultimate crisis hit about ten months after Sally started eating enough. She'd had plenty of emotional troubles during that time, but after the second month nothing but hunger sent her to the refrigerator anymore. When problems came, she just felt anxious, or sad, or mad, or worried, but she didn't binge. Not even a cookie. But this catastrophe at the ten-month mark wasn't like anything else she'd ever endured. The emotions it provoked were bigger and more overwhelming, and it shook her to the foundation: Sally's husband announced that he was leaving her and their three sons, ages four, three and eighteen months. He said he was in love with another woman.

Sally's husband worked as a freelance carpenter and Sally stayed at home with the boys, baby-sitting kids from the neighborhood in their apartment. Sally hadn't worked at an outside job since her second son was born. She knew the rent payments were two months late. Her husband hadn't found much work the six weeks before he dropped this bomb.

At first she was numb, then incredulous. Then she was furious, and after that, rageful. (Her husband got the rage part.) And at last, Sally was terrified. She went to the grocery store for milk and ended up buying pastries and chocolate bars and ice cream. Back home she laid them out on the table, determined to eat until she felt better. But two bites into the Hershey's bar, she burst into tears and couldn't eat anymore. "I'm even a failure at bingeing!" she wailed.

Sally could not binge. It wasn't physically possible for her anymore because she was too well fed. There was no empty vat to fill. She'd filled it in by eating so well every day for ten months. So Sally was left with her feelings. She sobbed and sobbed and finally she called a friend who came over to help.

"There's only one good thing about this whole mess," she choked out through her tears, confiding to her worried friend: "I can't binge anymore, no matter what. I just can't do it. I'm too full."

Sally weathered the storm very well indeed, and continued to take excellent care of her body's fuel needs. Slowly, she lost weight. In fact, over the next two years she lost a lot of weight. She looked good and she knew it. It wasn't just the weight. Her attitude toward herself and the world had changed. She had an attitude that showed—confident and strong. I'm sure I detected a glimmer of gloat in her face as she told me about the look on her ex-husband's face when they last met in court. This was almost two years after he left her.

"When I walked into the courtroom, he looked up but didn't recognize me and went on talking to his attorney," Sally recalls with a slight grin. "Then, when we all stood when the judge came in, he looked over and must have recognized me by deduction. When we sat down he pushed his attorney back in his chair to get a better look at me. I could see him out of the corner of my eye. I admit, I played it up to the max. I was dressed to the nines with makeup and hair to kill. I couldn't help taking the opportunity, you know, to get him back, just a little. Anyway, he just gawked like a schoolboy. He didn't look so hot. I almost felt sorry for him. It was gratifying.

"The thing that people need to understand about this program is this: when you get your eating straightened out, and stop starving yourself, much more than your diet is going to change. Your whole life changes in a way. I mean it. My entire life has changed because I finally learned to eat. I'm quite a different person. Ask anybody who knew me then and knows me now. I've changed!" she concludes.

• "THE MEDIA TELL YOU WHAT'S PERFECT, AND I WANTED TO LOOK LIKE THAT"—*Kelly T.*

The oldest child of a stockbroker and a realtor, Kelly developed unusually early and had completed the physical changes of puberty by age eleven. This wasn't a problem by itself, but Kelly was tall and big-boned and her best friends were short, prepubescent string beans. The discrepancy really bothered her. "One of the big things when you're that age," Kelly explains, "is fitting in—being like your friends. Otherwise you feel rejected because you're different. No one actually has to reject you. You just feel it." Teen magazines only made Kelly's struggle worse by reinforcing her body-image troubles. According to The Thin Ideal, she was clearly too curvy, too padded and too big.

Kelly asked her mother to make a doctor's appointment for her in order to get a diet to lose weight. Her mother protested because Kelly was obviously not overweight, but she made the appointment to satisfy her daughter's concerns, hoping the doctor would dissuade Kelly from dieting. It didn't happen. Kelly's weight was twelve pounds above the normal range for girls her height and age (probably because she was so athletic), and the doctor gave Kelly a 1,500-calorie diet and a list of foods to avoid. This no-no list included all junk foods, fatty meats and dairy products. So far so good. Kelly decided to strictly avoid these foods. But the thing she didn't consciously decide to do, but started doing anyway, was to go hungry.

Going without enough food and tolerating hunger wasn't really hard for Kelly for several reasons. She was extremely busy, so she didn't get much of a chance to dwell on her hunger. And she was an athlete. Her high physical activity level helped keep her consciousness of hunger under control. "Between my school schedule and athletics," she says, "I didn't have a chance to think about being hungry, but now, looking back, I was famished."

It took only a few weeks for Kelly's efforts to show, and people began to notice her more slender shape. In fact, just about everyone noticed. Her friends said things like, "You look great!" and "You're so skinny, what are you doing?" And Kelly was getting skinny. She admits now that her body had been OK before she lost weight, and now she sees that the standard to which she compared herself wasn't realistic for her. But she didn't know it then, so these comments meant a lot to her. She felt she finally fit in. Powerful stuff for a preteen.

Kelly's parents had become concerned by this time. Her eating had grown from a simple diet into an obsession. She was extremely rigid about the types of foods she was willing to eat, and virtually all of them were fat-free. If she stayed overnight with a friend, Kelly brought her own food, and she'd disappear during suppertime to run, she said, when there were family get-togethers. All this alarmed Kelly's parents, especially her mother.

There had been no significant dieting in her family, so Kelly's parents were confused about their daughter's strict dieting—what she now called "eating healthy." There was a family emphasis on sports and physical activity, but no talk of dieting or weight issues. Neither parent had ever dieted, nor had a weight problem. There had been no pressure at home on Kelly to look a certain way, no comments made about her weight, that is, until her mother accused her of looking too thin. Searching for a clue to her daughter's deepening troubles with food, Kelly's mother lost her patience when she read an article about eating disorders. Kelly had six of the ten symptoms listed under anorexia and possibly more. She made an appointment with the same doctor who had put Kelly on the diet in the first place.

At this point the battles between Kelly and her parents intensified. Accusations flew: "You look terrible—you've got to eat more food. Why don't you eat something normal for a change?" Kelly's little brother teased her, calling her a freak. Kelly says these darts made her feel guilty, but ultimately contributed to her determination to eat even less—sort of an "I'll show you who's in charge here" retaliation. The power struggles raged.

Kelly kept her doctor's appointment. She went because she was forced to go. She hadn't had a period in three months, although that didn't really bother her. It did bother her mother.

The physical exam revealed that Kelly had lost twenty-five pounds in five months since her first visit to the doctor. Her formerly muscular five-foot eight-inch frame was gaunt and bony at 123 pounds, and her eyes were big, round and bloodshot. The gray circles around them made her look old and tired. But Kelly denied that she was tired, hungry or sick. She insisted that she felt fine. Why didn't her parents just leave her alone? All she was doing was what a doctor had told her to do in the first place, so what was the big deal, anyway?

Kelly was referred to an eating disorders clinic. After the initial evaluation an eating disorders specialist met alone with her. "You're anorectic," she said bluntly. "Let's talk about it." This counselor was, according to Kelly, about fifty pounds overweight. "It really cut into her credibility," Kelly remembers.

The talking Kelly and her counselor did focused mainly on the power struggle between Kelly and her parents. Kelly now insists that this struggle had nothing to do with her developing an eating disorder. As she explains, "The power struggle could have made my anorexia worse because I got so mad at them for trying to tell me how to eat. Finally I decided to eat even less, to get back at them, but our fights didn't cause anything. They were the result of my determination not to have anyone interfere with my eating or not eating. The thing that got my anorexia started was this: I wanted to be thin like my friends. It was that goal that got it going and kept it going, right into the crazy time."

The "crazy time" Kelly refers to is the dead end she came to in her anorectic eating. She continued to lose weight during her "treatment" and became emaciated. She had also started abusing diuretics to get rid of the "bloated" feeling she had most of the time. At this point her diet had become extremely limited and she couldn't turn her self-starvation off. Some days she ate only an apple or a salad. Other days all she'd allow herself was a piece of no-fat bread. She sipped herbal tea to make her hunger more tolerable. She now admits that she was extremely hungry during this phase of her illness, but she never admitted it then, not to others and not to herself.

Although she kept regular appointments at the clinic, Kelly swears these meetings did nothing to influence her eating choices. If there was an effect, it was this: these visits made her even more determined to eat the way she wanted to eat because she felt that

the clinic was trying to take this right away from her. It seemed
that nothing could persuade her to eat more at this point. Kelly
had fallen into a dangerous place in food jail.

A year into her eating problems Kelly learned about the Naturally Thin concepts. But she didn't apply the principles to herself
because she couldn't see the Feast or Famine Cycle in her own
eating. She just never feasted, so she didn't count her chronic
famine as legitimate. Kelly never thought of her undereating as
famining. Ironically, her anorectic undereating was always cloaked
in her favorite "healthy eating" label.

"I never lost control of my eating because I was so determined
to lose weight, and when I'm determined, nothing can deter me,"
she explains. "It's my personality. I've never binged because I
wouldn't let myself, no matter how hungry I felt. No matter how
little I did eat, I always figured I was eating enough. You get in this
little world of your own and you can't see anymore. Everybody's a
threat to your way of handling this—and you're convinced in your
soul that it's not only the right way, it's the only way."

Kelly feels that the personality traits of determination and perfectionism make certain people more susceptible to anorexia.
Willpower is so strong and stubborn that it can overcome the instinct to survive. Kelly had it.

Ironically, the doctor who prescribed her original diet was the
one who helped Kelly begin to see her symptoms as danger signals. Kelly had a certain respect for this doctor since she had
taken her seriously the first time they met. And this doctor didn't
threaten or accuse her and never berated Kelly for the choices she
made. Instead, she persuaded Kelly to add foods to her diet, little
by little, for health reasons, of course. She also convinced Kelly
that the diuretics were backfiring, causing her to actually retain
fluids. Kelly slowly limited and then eliminated them.

Kelly's friends were supportive, too. They told her they were
worried about her and wanted to help. They also brought up the
subject of her eating disorder with great care, helping her look at
what she was doing to herself. Their gentle prodding helped support Kelly in the changes she was making. And very importantly,
they told Kelly how great she looked when she began to put on a
little weight, reinforcing her courage to change.

The Naturally Thin guidelines were a backup plan for Kelly, one
she didn't need or use until she had just started to gain weight.
When she contacted me, she had gained three pounds and was

worried. We went over the path she'd taken to anorexia, the
Famine Track. And we talked about the options for her—to continue to gain, gradually giving her body more and more power to
control her eating, or to retreat into starvation. She was terrified of
gaining too much weight and didn't know how to start without going out of control. I told her that this program was the antidote to
losing control of your eating. She said she understood that, but
she was still terrified.

The Naturally Thin principles were in place to provide Kelly
with the security of knowing that eating enough was the key to
her natural leanness—the ultimate vaccine against a life in food
jail. But she needed to know that she was about to gain some very
necessary weight—adaptive post-famine weight—and there was
no way around it if she wanted to get completely free.

Most of my coaching Kelly consisted of reminding her of these
principles and reassuring her that her body could do it. When her
weight began to increase back to normal, the most important decisions she made were to stop weighing herself and to wear bigger
clothes. Kelly gained weight for nearly a year, plateaued for five
months and then returned to her prediet weight over the next
twenty months.

"I still fear getting fat," she admits. "I have very heavy relatives
on my mom's side, and I take after that side of the family. When I
see a fat person on the street, it scares me. I think, I don't want to
ever look like that. And when I see real thin people, I want to look
like them—and better! I just have to keep my thinness ambition
under control and let my body control my eating."

When I asked Kelly what she thought caused eating disorders,
she responded quickly: "First the media tells you what's perfect, and
I wanted to look like that. It creates the standard for beauty in
America, and puts pressure on you to look a certain way. Then
peers because we all compare ourselves and there's always some-
body skinnier. Then personality and biology. Personality probably
influences which eating problem you'll get because only certain
types of people can stand to go hungry for long periods of time.
The ones who can, and are real ambitious about being superthin,
can get anorexia. It's easier than you might think. You get so subjective. Other kids get into bulimia because they lose it and binge.
Once you binge, you have to vomit because otherwise you'll get fat.
If I had ever binged, I would definitely have tried throwing up."

Kelly's a runner, soccer player and avid skier, and now she

knows that she has to eat well, and enough, in order to be an effective athlete. "I eat to perform," she explains. "If I don't do my part, my body can't do well, and I always want to do well, if not the very best." Her diet has developed into about eight "feedings" throughout the day—eaten whenever she's hungry. Because of her high activity level, and high complex-carbohydrate, low-fat diet, Kelly has to eat often—every one and a half to two hours. And she does. She figures she needs, and eats, close to 3,000 calories a day now, a figure she couldn't imagine a few years ago. "It's amazing the amount of food you can burn when you're naturally thin," she says with a smile.

• "I WAS ON AN ENERGETIC HIGH THAT LED ME STRAIGHT INTO HELL"—*Lisa P.*

Actress–model–TV host Lisa tells her story with excitement. "It's just amazing to me," she says, "that my body and I could get that offtrack and still find our way back to sanity."

The youngest daughter of Spanish immigrants, Lisa remembers a "skinny childhood." She and her whole family were always eating. Still a "stick" in high school, she didn't go through puberty until she was seventeen. There were plenty of dieters among her friends, but Lisa says she always thought dieting was too much work for her. As a cheerleader and athlete, she felt she had to eat plenty of food just to keep up with her high energy needs.

The first time Lisa ever thought she had gained weight was during her senior year, when she became depressed and her activity level decreased dramatically, but she says she was "too lazy" to do anything about it. These extra pounds were soon shed when she resumed her normal high-paced lifestyle.

Lisa had started modeling professionally as a junior in high school, but never told anyone because she thought it would label her. The year after she graduated from high school, she was finally free to model full-time. She decided to enroll in college full-time too, accepting a challenge from her dad. So Lisa's schedule was more frantic than ever, but she was happy—doing exactly what she wanted.

On an honor's scholarship at college, Lisa was under pressure to get very high grades in all her classes. She was taking eighteen credits—an ambitious full load. And her modeling career was taking off big time as she flew to three different cities a week between local jobs. These two careers, coupled with Lisa's serious asthma, began to take their toll. She began to lose weight.

"I was not trying to lose weight. I simply had no hunger at this time," Lisa explains. "I was simply too stressed to feel much of anything physical. I was on an energetic high."

Lisa's family noticed that she was getting way too thin and had dark circles under her eyes. Her mother confronted her, but Lisa brushed it off. "I'm just busy, Mom. Don't worry." But three months of this rat-race schedule—traveling, studying, modeling and very little sleep—were about to blow Lisa's life apart.

As her weight dropped other people—Lisa's agents and clients—noticed, too. And they liked what they saw—a thinner, a very thin Lisa. They often made comments when Lisa was on a job. She had to admit that she liked her new very thin look: "I liked being so thin—a size two! If I didn't eat I had more energy, and if I did eat at this point, my stomach got big."

It all came apart one morning. Lisa could not get up—literally. She could hardly move. Her body simply refused to take commands anymore, and her life came to a dead standstill. Her asthma kicked in severely and she didn't have energy for anything. She dropped out of college and told her modeling agency to take her off the schedule indefinitely. Lisa is frank about it: "I had a breakdown."

When she stopped her breakneck pace, Lisa's hunger was enormous and she started eating—large amounts of food often. She gained weight very quickly and seemed unable to stop herself until she was back up to her original weight. She explains: "I got so depressed and began to obsess about losing every pound I'd gained. My fear of never losing this weight became huge because I thought my career as a model would be over if I couldn't get it under control. I tried to control it by allowing myself to eat only once a day. Naturally I was starving, and ate these huge amounts of rich foods, but my body couldn't take it and then I began to throw it up. I wasn't forcing my body to throw up, my body was doing it by itself. I kept the weight on anyway."

Lisa admits now that this was a serious and crazy eating pattern, but back then she didn't care. Her mother did, though. She wrote to Lisa's aunt, who wrote to Lisa matter-of-factly: "You're anorectic and bulimic." "Deep down I knew," Lisa says, "but I thought, Oh crud—now they know." The secret was out.

At a family party during this time, Lisa ate all the icing on a very large birthday cake, besides a quart of ice cream. When she got home, she threw up as usual. That was when the thought first struck her, There is a problem here.

She now realizes: "I was in a trap, and I didn't have a clue about how to get out. I was still a size six, but I knew I couldn't hold my weight there. My face was puffy—bloated—the worst fear for a model.

"A friend who knew I was struggling with my weight told me about the Naturally Thin Program, and it just made sense to me. It explained everything I'd been through so far, as well as what I was going through now—post-famine feasting and weight gain. I knew I didn't have a choice—I had to do this—so I started eating, and overeating, with a vengeance. I wanted to gain as much as I had to and get it over with, but the food was still coming up. My body didn't seem to be ready at first, but gradually, the food stayed down and I gained. Knowing I'd have to fight my body the rest of my life if I didn't do this frightened me even more than weight gain."

Lisa called food her "medicine" during this phase, and she ate religiously whenever she was hungry, and sometimes when she was not. She actually hated eating after a while and wished she could just go hungry once, but she didn't. During this time she realized that she was eating like a normal person again—no obsessing, no bingeing, no cravings.

The tough part started when Lisa gained about fifteen pounds and then plateaued for eighteen months. This was the hardest time—the wait for the weight loss to begin—but wait she did.

"Coming out" as an overweight former model was Lisa's biggest emotional challenge. It marked the loss of her thin identity. She noticed old friends staring at her because of her weight. She noticed that men didn't notice her. She heard whispers, "Is that Lisa?" and she knew what they meant: Isn't it sad—she was a model. Concerned friends asked her if she was OK. Yep, she was OK. "These fifteen pounds were like a hundred pounds. I cried for four months," Lisa reflects.

Her need for support was greatest during this plateau. No one knew about Lisa's eating disorder except her mother, aunt and, eventually, me. Since her mom and aunt had no knowledge of Naturally Thin, Lisa called me.

LISA: Jean, I want someone to induce me to get this weight loss started.

JEAN: Lisa, I know you do, but your body has to do it, and it will. The wait is always hard.

LISA: I'm tempted to diet, but I know if I do I'll never be thin. What can I do to get this going?

JEAN: You can try cutting back on fats if you tolerate it, and exercise to firm up a bit. The exercise will make you feel better even though it won't make you lose weight.

"I bought bigger clothes instead." Lisa giggles. "Thinness was my idol. I got attention for it all the time. It was what I lived for. I hadn't been sympathetic to overweight people before this, although one of my close friends is heavy, but all that changed. All of a sudden I was like everybody else, and I didn't like it. My thinness had made me special. I missed it, but I knew I'd never be thin like I was before. I was different. Everything was different."

Lisa had become reclusive because of her weight gain, avoiding anyone who might recognize her from her "former life" as a thin model. But she found her way back, even while she was at her top weight.

The friend who had introduced Lisa to the program confronted her solitary lifestyle and she decided to audition for a TV job. She got it, even overweight. She also tried to model but was rejected. Lisa looked heavy on TV and she knew many old friends would see her. But it didn't matter anymore. She was learning to live with the extra weight, to go on with her life. And when her weight wasn't the center of her life anymore, Lisa says, the extra pounds slowly began to fall off. As they did, Lisa continued to eat freely and often, and many people commented about how she could eat so much and not be huge. She was actually getting smaller at that point.

Lisa returned to her model-thin figure and ended up with more work, especially in TV, than she'd ever had before. She even models swimwear, although her weight is a bit higher than it was before.

She says, "Food jail snuck up on me because I wasn't vigilant and I thought thinner must be better. I was so wrong. And I'm so relieved that I'll never have to go through that again!"

GETTING YOUR MONEY'S WORTH

Renee called me. "I've just got one question." "OK, shoot," I said.

"First let me tell you a little about me. I've been bulimic for over eight years. I've been to treatment twice, and in therapy full-time for a total of about six of the eight years. I figured that, in all, the treatment for my eating disorder has cost me $13,000, not counting what my insurance company paid. I have had no relief from this curse even with all this counseling.

"I found out about the Naturally Thin Program eight weeks ago today. I began to try to give my body more food more often at that time. I stopped going hungry completely by the second week or so. My last binge happened during that second week, and I purged then. I haven't binged or purged since. Not once. Not once. Here's my question: How do I get my money back?"

I sympathized with this woman in her frustration and anger. But I suggested that she was mistaken to think of her various therapies as a waste, simply because they hadn't cured her of bulimia. Just because her eating disorder was the problem that provoked her to seek treatment didn't mean that she hadn't gained from it in other ways. I suggested that she explore the different things that she had discovered from her work with professional counselors and therapists. I pointed out the fact that whether or not they had the answer to her problem, these well-educated, responsible and generally caring people had probably brought much to her life that she would have missed out on had she never sought help for her eating troubles.

UNDEREATERS ANOMALOUS

We've talked so much about membership in Overeaters Anonymous in this chapter that I feel I should clarify my position with the philosophy of this organization. Many of you have had an affiliation with OA simply because of its unique purpose and availability throughout the country.

The organization called Overeaters Anonymous is really misnamed. It should be called Undereaters Anomalous. The reason is simple: Overeating is not at the heart of the troubles from which the members suffer—undereating is. Overeating, as I have pointed out repeatedly in this book, is the symptom, a result of the problem, not the problem. The problem, as all of you well know by now, is undereating—eating late, going hungry, eating too little, skipping meals, eating poor-quality food, food avoidance, dieting—all based on the common fear of fatness and consequent fear of food in our culture.

Three

Helping Others Break Out and Stay Out of Food Jail

CHAPTER 8

Living Outside Jail: Food Friendly and Naturally Thin

The biases about weight problems are so rampant among professionals, including many obesity researchers, that it's no wonder the masses still see food as the enemy of lean bodies. One researcher on the forefront of news about obesity is Thomas Wadden, Ph.D. Dr. Wadden pretty well sums up the approach that scientists in this field have taken for over four decades. Discussing obesity, he says: "Its remedy seems so simple. People need to eat less and exercise more . . . Only recently have health professionals begun to appreciate obesity's alarming prevalence, its heterogenous etiology and its refractoriness to treatment."*

What that last sentence says, basically, is this: The scientific community is just beginning to wake up to the ever more obvious fact that the time-honored eat-less, exercise-more treatment for overweight doesn't make fat people thin. In fact, the more we try this approach, the more fat people we seem to have! No, it looks as if weight problems are just a bit more complicated than that.

Four years after making this statement, Dr. Wadden and four colleagues conducted a comprehensive five-year study assessing the influence of behavior modification on weight loss accomplished by dieting. The purpose of the study was to demonstrate

*Thomas A. Wadden, "Treatment of Obesity in Adults," *Innovations in Clinical Practice: A Source Book* 4 (1985): 127.

that behavior modification was the missing ingredient in long-term weight-loss (by dieting) success. In other words, this study was designed to show that teaching people to change their behavior regarding food could make weight loss produced by undereating permanent. But this is what was concluded at the end of the study: "Weight regain continued at the 5-year follow-up, at which time there was not even a hint of the effectiveness of behavioral treatment."* To translate, by the end of the five-year study, it was crystal clear that behavior modification had absolutely no beneficial effect on the 95-plus percent long-term failure rate of dieting. He went on to recommend that investigators prove that losing weight and gaining it back was better for people than just staying fat. More recent research has suggested that staying at a stable weight, even overweight, may be better for most people than weight fluctuations, even within normal limits.

The treatment of obesity in our country today is archaic, reflecting caveman-level thinking of the most simplistic nature. It's no wonder we are stuck at best, and causing more and more weight problems, health complications and eating disorders at worst. Besides the serious medical repercussions of obesity (and who knows whether these ill effects are not really related to intermittent famines?) and the terrible loss of energy and talent that results from our diet-crazed culture, the saddest consequence of this malevolent path is the epidemic of eating disturbances that it has created, particularly among young people.

And who among the professionals are the guilty ones? Many physicians and scientists who research obesity are guilty of promoting a popular treatment that has never proven to be effective in the long run, but may even be physically damaging. But not all physicians and researchers bear responsibility for the continued promotion of the eat-less diet approach. Some physicians refuse to recommend calorie-limited diets anymore, focusing instead on diet quality. But without an understanding of the necessity of an adequate calorie intake and sensitivity to hunger cues, this stance is largely unhelpful. There is just too much "eat less" publicity out there, keeping people locked in the Cycle.

Some researchers in the field are genuinely seeking answers,

*Thomas A. Wadden, Juliet A. Sternberg, Kathleen A. Letizia, Albert A. Strunkard, Gary D. Foster, "Treatment of Obesity by Low Calorie Diet, Behavior Therapy, and Their Combination," *International Journal of Obesity* 13 (1989): 39–46.

but most of their studies involve new ways to suppress the appetite (anti-eat pills) or biochemical interference with fat deposition (anti-fat pills). No one appears to be very interested in the glaring fact that bodies do not tolerate undereating as a lasting method for weight control or the reasons that bodies store fat in the first place. No, the "pros" are all apparently filled with the presumptions of the age.

The bias these professionals bring from the culture unfortunately seeps into their thinking, often contaminating their research interpretation and conclusions. Some are overtly malevolent toward overweight people, assigning to them character defects that must, they say, account for their resistance to treatment. These researchers are so frustrated by their failure to find real answers that, in the end, they put the problem on their clients or subjects in order to excuse themselves. Their faulty attitudes, unfortunately, find their way into their communications with the public, adding potency to popular prejudices about the overweight. These attitudes also promote much misfocused determination in those who already fear weight gain, making them even more vulnerable to eating disturbances.

THE POPCORN STUDY

One of the best examples of research bias I've seen involved a study of popcorn eaters at a frightening movie. This study was capsulized in *Reader's Digest,* the most widely read magazine in the world. In this study, the researchers hypothesized that overweight people would be more likely to eat in response to upsetting emotions than people of normal weight—the "psychological theory of obesity." So a group of overweight people and a group of normal-weight people were given premeasured bags of popcorn and sent to see a scary movie. They started out with the same amounts of popcorn, and after the movie, bags were remeasured. Guess what they discovered? The people who were overweight ate more popcorn than those who were of normal weight. You don't say.

The researchers concluded that their hypothesis was correct, that people who are overweight eat more when they have upsetting emotions than normal-weight people. Right. No one ever determined, in this "study," just who ate what before the popcorn and movie started. It's a well-known fact that most overweight people are trying to limit their food intake throughout the day so they won't get any fatter. So their normal resting state is underfed or hungry. Not so with normal-weight people—they eat more freely and their normal resting state is more satisfied. It looks to me as if the scary movie had nothing to do with how much popcorn anybody ate. Overweight people are simply *hungrier* than their thin counterparts because of their tendency to undereat whenever they can. People who are well fed don't usually eat much popcorn or other extra food. And perhaps the overweight subjects in the study felt permission to eat the popcorn freely, something that they look for to let their diet guard down.

At any rate, doesn't it look as if this study is trying to prove that fat people have emotional problems that make them eat so much? You bet it does. It seems to have been set up to prove a popular tenet of our culture: Fat people really are emotional jellyfish who can't control their feelings or their eating. Boy, oh boy, you sure don't want to be in this group!

It looks as if we don't have enough disrespect for overweight people already or fear of becoming like them—we've got to conduct studies to prove that our rejection of them is based on proven facts, despite the clear findings of other research that obese people do not suffer from any more psychological problems than nonobese people. What they do suffer from is a culture that summarily rejects them for being overweight, and if that doesn't make most of them neurotic or paranoid, then they're a pretty psychologically hardy lot.

The rejection that overweight people universally experience in our culture is precisely what people with disturbed eating suffer from, too—intense, even pathological fear of being overweight. This is not a neurotic fear; it seems to be proportionate to the potential consequences at stake. This fear causes weight gain in many dieters by interfering with regular adequate food intake. But in others, adaptive weight gain is obstructed by powerful counter-adaptation tactics designed to keep the intensified appetite controlled or the food absorption limited. People with eating struggles are really quite sane in their original purpose—avoiding obesity—but the war they wage with their bodies often leads to insane methods of coping.

But wait, some of these "insane" methods are actually being taught—by professionals. I kid you not. Recently, because of concern over the growing disrepute of food, the American Institute of Food and Wine decided to go on the offensive in supplanting the reputation of food in our culture. (This fact, in itself, is pitiful evidence of the problem to which I allude.) No one even questions as bizarre the need for food to be "sold" as a positive commodity. The AIFW hired the president of the American Dietetic Association to soothe the nation's food concerns, chiefly through the media. This top dietitian's job, it seems, is to reassure people that it really is OK to eat food, at least some foods, at least sometimes. This job gets tricky fast.

And it really does, what with the cholesterol fears and the pesticide fears and hormone worries and cancer risks and the absolute necessity of weight control. So, what does an expert nutritionist offer in the way of reassurance to our starving, fearful masses? You won't believe it. While she is pointing out the fact that, because of their fear of food, most women are trying not to eat, her explanation for why these women then eat an entire bag of cookies is the guilt they feel after eating just one. This reflects the ever-popular "overeating is emotionally induced" theory that pervades treatment centers for the eating disordered. Sweets and fatty foods, she suggests, creep mysteriously into the diets of the overconscientious eating-avoidant. She calls this "irrational elimination of some behaviors but compensating with other irrational choices." Does that make sense? But this isn't the worst part, not by far.

Her "golden rule" of good eating is (drumroll please): portion control. Here we go again, right back to the heart and soul of dieting: measure your cornflakes. And I suppose this golden rule is supposed to reassure all of us out here in food-phobic dietland that food really is safe—in very limited, carefully controlled and premeasured amounts. Makes you feel much better about food, doesn't it? But the best is yet to come.

This dietitian, who is at the very top of her field as head of the American Dietetic Association (where information about many of our standard fears originates), offers a list of tips for making meals "more fun," yet staying within reasonable calorie and fat limits (of course). Let me share a few of her ideas with you.

1. When dining out, tell the waiter not to bring bread and butter until the meal is served.

Well, I haven't discovered how this little trick is going to add fun to your dinner out, especially if you're starved when you get to the restaurant and can't converse until you have a few harmless calories in your tummy. Since I became naturally thin over ten years ago, I often insist that the bread be brought immediately when I eat out. That's when I need it—not later when the table is chock-full of dinner and I have all the food I can possibly eat besides the bread. Eating bread appeases my appetite, and that's what I want it to do so I can hold a conversation and won't need to stuff myself later.

Obviously, this expert is working under the old "out of sight, out of mind" rule, as if bread had some evil power to provoke your lust for excess calories. The reason bread is at the table before the meal is to satisfy the uncomfortable too-hungry feeling of many diners. Let's not discourage this humane custom, nor the waiters who uphold it.

2. Ask for a take-home container when the meal is served so you can put aside the amount you want to take home.

The implication here is this: Quick, get most of this delicious food off your plate and packed away in an opaque Styrofoam doggie bag so you won't go off the deep end and eat all of it in one sitting. You can't trust yourself to stop when you should (after eating a scientifically determined portion, calculated in a laboratory, based on average metabolic rates of male rats in shoe box mazes with negative activity levels). Nope, better save it for later, when you'll feel too anxious and/or guilty to eat it because of the double hot fudge brownie delight you picked up on your way home.

It does perplex me just how this storage container usage could add to my fun while dining out, not to mention my date's.

3. At home, immediately freeze portions before eating a whole batch of anything.

I actually know of someone who tried this. She, too, was afraid of multi-portions of food and separated them out into less threatening little bundles, freezing them, thereby rendering them relatively tasteless and consequently harmless. The only hitch she ran into was the exposure she had to the rest of the contents of the freezer. Whenever she'd go for a premeasured, less threatening portion of whatever she had made, say, spaghetti, she'd come across the ice cream, too—and not carefully separated into harmless bundles. Now, sometimes she could get the little baggie of pasta out and quickly slam the freezer door, hardly noticing the ice cream, which, by the way, was not rendered relatively tasteless by freezing. But the frozen portions always took awhile, ten minutes or so, to cook, and, more often than not, she'd have scooped out several generous "portions" of ice cream for herself by the time her pasta was on a plate before her. By then, however, she usually wasn't in the mood for spaghetti, and just continued with the ice cream until she was full and/or disgusted with herself.

Perhaps this frozen portion plan works better for others.

Send testimonials to my attention.

4. When buying bread, put two-slice packets in the freezer so in the morning you're not tempted to toast four slices and slather them with marmalade.

You have got to be putting me on here. No, this is really a serious "tip" from a registered dietitian who is trying to reassure the public about the safety of eating food. We are not talking about fatty taco chips and guacamole dip or corn dogs and pie à la mode. We're talking about bread! Does this sound a little compulsive to you? Should our freezers be full of little two-pack "safety slices" and premeasured mini-portions of food, all silently protecting us from overindulging? Think of this message, especially in light of what it's supposed to be accomplishing, and it's quite preposterous! But this fear-driven obsessive food control is something else, too—it's a tragedy. It's feeding our nation's growing obesity and eating disorders problems, which are already at epidemic levels.

EXTERNAL CONTROL

I think I know what this professional, and others like her, are getting at. They're trying to address the exaggerated appetite that undereaters experience, that requires enormous external control to keep in line. If this woman really does abide by the tips she suggests, then she has an eating disorder. She is undoubtedly on the Feast or Famine Cycle. Natural, body-controlled eaters don't have to work that hard to eat the right amount of food when they get hungry. Their bodies tell them the right amount, and they are always listening.

The idea of trying to control eating from outside the body is a basic tenet of dieting. One well-known external control tactic is fondly known as the "little plate" trick. To fool the eater's perception of a portion of food, the use of a smaller plate has been recommended for decades. The same amount of food looks larger, the smaller the plate it's placed on. And another tip like it suggests that you chew food fifty times before swallowing it, thereby convincing your mouth that you're eating more food, the more you chew. The only problem with these tricks is this: The body won't be fooled. Undereating can't be fixed by adjusting perceptions of amounts of food eaten. No, the only way to really fix undereating is to eat more food. I know it's scary, but it's so.

A doctor from the Albert Einstein College of Medicine in New York has made some specific recommendations for controlling food intake, too. He suggests using opaque containers for leftovers in the refrigerator so you won't be able to see the contents. This is along the same lines as asking the waiter not to bring bread before the meal. See no food, eat no food. Then he adds that you can unscrew the bulb in the refrigerator so none of the food can be seen, at least without a flashlight. And another suggestion for giving your body the false impression that you really are eating enough is to use baby utensils. This has double benefits in forcing slow eating, plus making the consumption of a whole portion very difficult without unlimited time at lunch. Either way, I don't know if your clients, dates or friends would be much impressed.

When I share these suggestions at Naturally Thin Seminars, audiences laugh wildly. They laugh because, in the context of the Naturally Thin principles, these tactics look completely absurd. No one in her right mind would behave like this! And they laugh because many of them have tried these things, and similar tactics, to outsmart their hungry bodies. And how has it worked?

For most veteran dieters, some of whom have eaten from dog dishes and garbage pails, opaque leftover containers just aren't going to keep them from eating and, when their bodies take over following a diet, overeating. No, tiny utensils and baggie-sized portions and keeping the bread out of sight just aren't going to do the trick. The sad thing is, we keep searching for new diet tricks to keep us from eating as much as we need when the ones we know about fail us. Just look at the cover topics of women's magazines for new diet tips. There's a list or two every month. But there is no magic diet trick—only one simple solution. And that we are unwilling to do because of our ignorance and fear.

Professionals and diet companies alike have come up with

dozens of creative methods for keeping their clients away from food. Some tactics, like the ones just described, border on insanity and should positively insult normal, self-respecting people. But often they don't because people have been so indoctrinated about the importance and even the necessity of these gimmicks to keep our eating in line that they no longer recognize how silly they are.

Other methods for managing the control of food intake are more serious because they have the stamp of medical authority on them. These include "medically supervised" liquid fast and other very low calorie diets, calorie-restricted prescription diets like diabetic diets and other food-limited diets to promote weight loss for medical reasons. When doctors tell you to do something, somehow you feel it must be right, and usually it is. But sometimes it isn't.

BUT I'M HUNGRY!

Joleen came to see me when she was eighteen. She'd been diabetic since birth and had no trouble with her diet or insulin regulation until at thirteen she learned to check her blood sugar by testing her blood. Joleen started to control her eating based on her blood-sugar test results. She became very anxious whenever it was too high and wouldn't eat, even if she was hungry, because eating would make it even higher. Going hungry like this gradually led her first to the Feast or Famine Cycle and then to the FeaFam Cycle. She was diagnosed with bulimia at fourteen.

Bulimia is serious in anyone, but it can be fatal in a diabetic. At a treatment center for bulimia, Joleen learned all the psychological reasons for her eating disorder, including the notion that she was rebelling against having diabetes. There were family issues, too—her dad was a doctor, and that was supposed to be at the heart of her power struggle.

A diabetic team worked very hard with this young woman for the next four years, trying to get her eating and insulin dose stabilized. Joleen complained almost constantly of feeling hungry. Her caregivers told her that her hunger was a symptom of her eating disorder, that her 1,800-calorie diabetic diet was adequate for her weight and activity level. Besides, she was a bit overweight, having gained twenty pounds in treatment. Finally, after begging her dietitian again for more food, Joleen was referred to me.

I knew Joleen was hungry, really hungry. She'd been seriously underfed during her two years of bulimia and then she'd been on a calorie-controlled eating regimen, afraid to increase her intake for fear her diabetes would get out of control. Her hunger was still exaggerated from her famines; moreover, I wasn't convinced that 1,800 calories was enough for her anyway. I told her I believed she was really hungry for more food because she needed to eat more. She was relieved that someone believed it wasn't all in her head.

With the cooperation of her doctor and diabetic team, Joleen started eating more food based on her hunger signals. Of course, her insulin had to be increased, too, and her blood sugars watched very carefully. Gradually, Joleen's hunger was satisfied and her weight went up about five pounds. She felt much, much better in general, so her team voted to continue allowing her body more say in her diet. Gradually, Joleen's appetite dropped down, and her blood sugar came down closer to normal limits than they'd been before she started eating more. She lost weight. Her need for insulin stabilized.

Joleen always ate only the best-quality foods in balance because of her diabetes, and gradually she let her body have almost complete control of how much to eat and when. Guess what? She isn't hungry anymore.

Although this is unorthodox (and dangerous without medical supervision), the same principles at work here can lead anyone out of food jail. Joleen's recovery is especially significant because she's been rescued from the many complications and risks of eating disorders, which are grave when combined with diabetes. Her medical team is to be commended for their willingness to go along with Joleen's insistence on trying something new. They may have started with the typical prejudices, but they were open and consequently able to help this desperate young woman to a much healthier eating pattern.

WHERE ARE WE GOING?

I noticed, in a women's magazine, a special list of nutritional terms that every woman should know. Here's a partial list of the terms that were defined:

sugar-free
dairy-free
calorie-free
no-calorie
low-calorie
no-fat
low-fat
light
lean
less filling
less than low-fat
lower than low-low-fat
the lowest fat possible but not as tasteless as completely no-fat
so low-fat that under a microscope you can't detect a fat cell
cardboard food—no calories, no fat, no sugar, no taste—won't
   do anything for you
exercise morsels—workout substitutes for negative calorie eating

If we take the current trend in food avoidance to its natural conclusion, we should simply put warning labels on all foods that contain any calories whatsoever. This label could read:

> CAUTION! This product contains calories that cause weight gain and consequent social discrimination. DO NOT USE this product if you want to be thin enough to be accepted or admired. Regular use of this product may impair your ability to have any kind of decent life.

The "safe" foods left would include black tea, black coffee, diet pop, sugar-free powdered drinks and water. You'd never have to worry about your weight if you just stuck with this "safe" list. Of course, you'd have to go with the natural water-processed decaf on the coffee and tea, and there is that aspartame controversy to consider with the sugar-free products. And, oh, yes, I read that the dyes in powdered drinks could be used to restain Alexander Calder's outdoor sculptures, so they might not be that easy on your digestive system. Guess we're down to water. Now water's safe for sure, except for the high levels of chlorine and trace minerals that can build up in your, was that the liver or the kidneys? And isn't all that carbonation in bottled spring water being linked to gas problems?

Do you see where we're headed? Maybe I'm stretching the point a bit, but it deserves to be stretched. We have to stop this war on food and declare, instead, a war on the fear of food. Quality foods need not be labeled with warnings, although poor-quality food might bear a caution, but diet products definitely deserve to be called DANGEROUS.

I can see it now, in big letters on every can of that famous weight-loss "shake":

> CAUTION: Use of this product is likely to lead to weight gain, obesity, dangerous weight fluctuations, appetite-control problems, bingeing, cravings for sweet and fatty foods, preoccupation with food, urge to eat without discernable hunger, emotional overeating, bulimia, anorexia, food addiction and compulsive overeating; DO NOT USE this or any other diet product without the advice and consent of your heath care provider.

We might make food more user friendly by reminding people that the good old four food groups are designed to help them keep variety and balance in their diets. Coupled with lower fat guidelines, all they need to know is this: If they're eating enough to keep up with their bodies' fuel needs, they won't have trouble with sweets or overeating. If they aren't eating enough, they're going to have trouble staying with quality food and moderate portions. There it is in a nutshell. I know, there'll be protests because I haven't told you whether frozen yogurt is a quality food or not, but I'll just bet you can figure it out. (If you need—I mean need—to eat frozen yogurt, you're not eating enough.)

The technology that's gone into assessing food value nowadays is unbelievable. We know more about calorie contents, and percentage of calories from fat, and total daily dietary fat allowances and carbohydrates split up into simple sugars, unprocessed sugars and corn syrup–type sugars than ever before. Guess what? Most of it's unnecessary. In fact, I believe this excessive food technology both reflects and promotes the anxiety we have about food and eating in our culture. We are obsessed with eating right, with controlling our food intake at ridiculous levels. And we are getting fatter, succumbing to a host of weight-related troubles, as our attempts to control our eating grow.

WHERE THE FOOD SUPPLY IS UNCERTAIN

Jane Brody, the well-known nutrition expert and author, has contributed more to food friendliness than most, but she, too, sometimes leans toward the "we are fat simply because we have too much food" attitude. For example, although she gets close to the adaptation idea here, she is unaware of the typical patterns of eating avoidance among overweight people: "They [overweight people] are actually better suited to survival than those who can't seem to put on an ounce—better suited, that is, *if they lived in a place where the food supply was uncertain* [italics mine]: feast one day, famine the next. Fortunately, or unfortunately, our food supply in late twentieth-century America is hardly uncertain."*

What Ms. Brody is missing here is absolutely critical. Food supply is not about food in the grocery store or at the nearby fast-food restaurant. The "food supply" for each body is dependent upon the eating behavior of the individual. If a person doesn't eat because she is dieting or too busy or whatever, the food supply for her body *is* uncertain, just as it would be if she lived in a part of the world with unpredictable food rations. We have to get over the presumption that just because we have an abundance of food, we must be getting an abundance to eat. Most of us are not getting enough to eat at the right times, and that is the heart of the problem.

If there is plenty of food in our country, as Ms. Brody correctly suggests, but there are scores of young women, especially, who develop mysterious ritual-laden obsessive behaviors regarding their food intake, isn't it safe to assume that something must be terribly wrong with these women mentally to cause such symptoms? It's been safe so far. In fact, on account of the obvious mental symptoms that many people with anorexia do develop, it's

*Jane Brody, *Jane Brody's Good Food Book* (New York: W. W. Norton, 1985), 188.

been deemed positively "factual"—that is, believed and taught as fact. But what happens when a theory like this becomes such a popularly held "truth"? The Salem witch-hunts come to mind.

WHAT DID YOU LEARN IN TREATMENT?

Monica sat cross-legged in my office, composed, tall and very, very thin. She told me that her troubles had started eleven years earlier, when she was seventeen. At that time she was admitted to treatment for anorexia.

I asked her what she had learned in treatment. "Nothing, really," was her reply, but when I pressed her to look more carefully, she discovered that she had learned a great deal.

Monica shared what she had learned: that her eating disorder was emotional. She learned that she took her feelings out on her body by refusing to eat. She learned that these powerful feelings—whatever they were—were interfering with her ability to feed herself like a normal person. And she learned that her eating disorder was her way of trying to control her life, which felt out of control during adolescence. Monica was still trying to figure out what feelings and control issues were keeping her trapped in anorexia when she came to see me.

I asked Monica why she had started starving herself in the first place. "My emotions, I guess," she shot back. I asked her to think it through again. What was the very first reason she could remember for trying to limit her eating? A knowing smile came over her face as she admitted, "I didn't like how I looked. That's it—the whole story. I didn't like my body and I wanted to change it. It was downhill from there."

And now, eleven years down a rocky road later, Monica is still afraid to eat because she's still afraid she'll gain weight and she still can't bear the thought of being fat. I don't blame her. She had learned one big thing in treatment—that she was emotionally screwed up. But it was a lie.

Therapists and doctors are indoctrinating people who have eating disorders with misbeliefs about themselves that are not only unhelpful, but can actually cripple them further. The common beliefs about emotional problems and eating disturbances have never been proven as cause/effect. They just show up together often enough, and because of a desperate need to make sense out of behavior that appears irrational on the surface, excited therapists jump to all kinds of conclusions that help them explain why people with eating problems behave the way they do. Then they indoctrinate their clients with these ideas, sharing superstitions with them as if they were facts. And their clients are just as eager to understand their own sick eating behavior as they, so they believe the theories offered. After all, these are experts!

Treatment center professionals explain to clients and their families, over and over again, that anorectics, bulimics, compulsive overeaters and food addicts all have tremendous emotional struggles that are manifested in their eating behavior. These ideas have been circulating for so long that everyone accepts them as unquestionable truth. This is irresponsible and even dangerous. Coupled with ignorance of the role of undereating in pathological eating patterns, it accounts for the miserable long-term recovery rate for people who seek treatment for eating disorders through available sources.

Monica says she wants to be free of her eating disorder forever. Although she is afraid, she is willing to make the necessary changes to move toward freedom. What will it take for her to get well?

PREREQUISITES FOR SUCCESS

People with eating disorders need certain qualities if they are going to get well. By "well" I mean having a normal relationship with food and with their bodies: cured. Here are the main characteristics I've observed in people who recover from eating disturbances by the Naturally Thin principles:

1. a deep belief in the principles of adaptation
2. a secure understanding that their symptoms have resulted from their undereating efforts
3. realization that their undereating efforts have resulted from their rational fear of being overweight in a culture that openly discriminates against overweight people, especially women

4. determination to get out of food jail no matter what they have to do
5. willingness and ability to face their fears of food, and weight gain, by eating more food when they get hungry, eventually letting go of most intellectual controls
6. ability to gradually let go of old, rigidly held beliefs and behaviors
7. recognition of personal vulnerabilities in eating and body image
8. motivation to work hard for recovery
9. perseverance

Clearly, it takes some serious personal strength to pull yourself out of food jail. I've never seen a weakling do it. But then, I have found that many people with eating problems are anything but weak. On the contrary, some seem to be the most determined people in the species. Their chances of getting well seem to be enhanced by the same qualities that helped set them up for eating troubles.

The two goals of the Naturally Thin eating program are:

1. a normal relationship with food
2. a normal relationship with your body

What exactly are we getting at here? What does "normal" mean? Normal eating is really simple: eating in response to physical cues without anxiety, fear, guilt or conflict. A normal relationship with food is easygoing. When you have one, food is nice but it's no big deal. You like to eat, but you don't think about it unless you're hungry.

Little kids are almost always body-controlled eaters. They wouldn't think of ignoring their hunger, and they don't care what time it is or when they ate last. They have no anxiety, fear, guilt or conflict about eating when they're hungry—that is, until misguided grown-ups teach them these unhappy feelings by imposing their food phobias on them.

This happened to Bella, a kindergartner whose height and weight were taken as part of her school screening tests. The nurse who recorded these statistics frowned and shook her head at the scale as she motioned for Bella's mother to speak with her privately.

The nurse said: "She's in the 80th percentile weight-wise. Did you know that?" (She did not wait for an answer.) "And her height is only in the 65th. Because of this discrepancy between the percentiles, with her weight 15 percent higher, you'd better start cutting down on her fat intake, no sweets or fried foods—ever. And is she active?" (Again she didn't wait for an answer.) "She should be active at least forty-five minutes daily—bicycling, running, jumping rope, whatever. Cut back on TV. That usually helps."

This nurse knew nothing of Bella's diet or physical activities. She assumed, from the discrepancy between her height and weight percentile scores, that Bella must be "overweight" and inclined to become more so. But to look at this little girl, you'd never suspect anything of the sort. She had a lovely, well-proportioned body—quite muscular—and not a hint of too much padding. Besides, her diet was very good—not perfect—but certainly balanced and healthy. Fortunately, Bella's mother sought some objective counsel before changing her daughter's routine or sharing this nurse's concerns about her weight with Bella. But what potential destruction this story represents to the millions of kids who are set up for eating worries by overly concerned and misguided adults!

Kids are natural-born eaters, and adults should be, too. We have to stop trying to teach children that food is hazardous, that going hungry is a good thing, and that physical activity must be done like a homework assignment. Instead, we'd better work on one main area where kids' nutrition is concerned: making good food available to them whenever they get hungry. Then adults can even learn about normal eating from kids.

I was accused once, by a friend with whom I was traveling, of being preoccupied with food, bringing it up every time I got hungry. And he was right. Every single time I got hungry I would tell him I needed to get something to eat. He would go six or eight hours without even mentioning food, so my every two- or three-hour interruptions must have seemed annoying. But he is forty pounds overweight and I am naturally thin. People who have a normal relationship with food seek food when they get hungry, and people with an unhealthy relationship with food often don't even know when they're hungry until they're starving.

So what's a normal relationship with your body? Like the relationship with food I just described, a healthy relationship with your body is marked by acceptance. You don't have to totally love every aspect of your physique to be in harmony with it. You do have to be relaxed about it so that it doesn't interfere with your life—your thinking, your choices, your eating behavior.

Body image that has been distorted by the standards of the culture and the bizarre patterns of eating disturbances can take a long time to mend. Years after eating behavior has normalized, some continue to struggle with accepting their bodies, and suffer from distortions in their perception of their physical selves. These people sometimes have to protect themselves against things that trigger their anxiety about their bodies. The most common culprits here are:

1. knowing their weight
2. clothes that are too small
3. comments from others about their bodies
4. overexposure to The Thin Ideal
5. exposure to diet information

HOW FLAT IS A DEAD STOMACH?

Judy's parents were both on the heavy side, and she was determined to remain svelte with strict diet and exercise routines. She had suffered a bout with anorexia, but increased her eating when she stopped having her periods because she knew that was "the danger signal." Now she never missed her seven-day-a-week workouts and swore she could tell if she did. "My stomach pooches out when I miss, and my husband teases me that I look pregnant, so I can't." Then she explained that her mother had a very big stomach and Judy "knew" it was so big because she didn't exercise.

Judy's workout schedule was fine for her until she got sick. It started out as a little cold, so she didn't think anything of continuing her ninety-minute routine. But when she developed chills and a fever she cut her time back to an hour, just to be on the safe side. That's what she said, anyway.

When Judy was diagnosed with pneumonia she asked her doctor if she could keep working out. He was stunned. She took three days off, and when she started up again she had such severe chest pain that she had her husband take her to the emergency room. Hospitalized for four days, Judy was referred to a psychologist by her doctor, and it came out in their conversations that her main motive for compulsive exercise was to avoid her husband's jabs. She decided that it might be better for her to accept the fact that she had inherited a little tummy bulge, tell her hubby to keep his comments to himself and cut back to four 45-minute workouts a week, thereby keeping herself on the planet a normal number of years.

IF YOU WANT IT YOU CAN HAVE IT, BUT NOBODY CAN GET IT FOR YOU

I've noticed something interesting in working with people who suffer from eating problems. It's a simple thing and generally applies to other problems. Those who want to get well, and are ready to do what it takes, and do it, do get well. And people who aren't ready, or won't do what it takes, don't, even if they say they really want to. I am confident that the biggest factor that separates one group from the other is the ability to let go of The Thin Ideal in order to learn to eat enough. Those who remain locked in their phobia of weight gain (even if they are already overweight) cannot break through to body-controlled eating. Their fear paralyzes them. Their desire to be free is sincere, I am sure, but they are locked in food jail, at least for now. But the ones who are ready, do the work and face the fear, well, you can only admire them for their courage.

Those I've known who do recover rarely require a lot of help from me. In fact, dozens of them contact me only after they are completely well, sharing their stories in order to encourage others. Sometimes other people, in a panic, will ask for support, or encouragement that they're on the right track, but usually no more than that. They don't ask me to hold their hands or do it for them. They know I can't, just as well as I do. They usually have the attitude, I got myself into this mess, and I must get myself out. They are so right.

But short of hand-holding, how can you get the support you may need, the kind of encouragement that will help you through the crisis points that come for many who are in jail? Deliberately, that's how. You must anticipate your need for support so that you'll be less likely to slip back into old eating controls for security.

There are two places to get support: personal friends and professional "friends." Both avenues offer groups that are especially helpful if everybody is trying to win freedom from food jail by the Naturally Thin principles. It won't help to go to a group like OA because OA doesn't believe in what you're doing—they think food is the problem and they don't think freedom from food jail is possible for "food addicts."

Personal friends, as we've discussed, have to know what you're doing in order to be helpful. It's a plus if the friend is naturally thin, or trying to get back to normal eating herself by Naturally Thin principles. Therapists must respect your approach, too, or you may be persuaded by their bias about emotional causes. Even if you share your plan with a professional counselor, you are likely to get some input about your emotional problems whether you want it or not. He or she just can't help it. So choose a pro for backup carefully.

DON'T LEAVE HOME WITHOUT WHAT?

While you're in the process of seeking support for getting your eating back to normal, pack one extra item in your lunch pail: this book. You never know when you may get sideswiped by a comment, photo, model or mirror. One "friend" you can always count on to give you a booster shot of honest feedback about your eating fears is in your hands right now. Nothing out there will tell it to you straight—the whole fascinating story about eating problems— like this book. Some say that just having the book around helps remind them and protect them from the onslaught of The Thin Ideal message coming at them from everywhere.

Mark up the book. Curl the pages. Use color-coded bookmarks. Highlight it. Photocopy pages you need on your bathroom mirror. Tear a chapter out that you need to reread and reread and reread. Use it, abuse it, but get the principles into your head. You'll feel better the worse your book looks.

HEALTH ISSUES TO CONSIDER

Getting well isn't always a smooth road health-wise. The havoc that eating disturbances can wreak on a body takes time and lots of right eating to remedy. Many, perhaps most, people who endeavor to break out of food jail by this method do so without any medical aid whatsoever. The process is necessarily gradual and slow, so bodies get ample time to readapt to the changes without anything getting too out of whack. But sometimes I recommend that a person get medical supervision, just in case. Here are the situations that warrant at least an initial physical exam and perhaps ongoing supervision by a doctor and/or a psychiatrist:

1. anyone with an acute/dangerous eating disorder (see Chapter 9, page 236.)
2. a person with any eating problem plus a chronic medical or psychiatric condition (diabetes, heart disease, mental disorder, ulcer, colitis, on prescription medication, etc.)
3. anyone with an eating disturbance and a history of serious depression
4. any pregnant woman with an eating disturbance
5. an abuse victim who has disturbed eating
6. anybody on nonprescription (street) drugs with an eating disturbance

OBSTACLES TO PROGRESS

Current methods for managing our weight would have us wary of eating and dependent on formal exercise programs if we are to stay thin. These approaches stem from the same beliefs that gave us the notoriously ineffective obesity treatment methods—that eating too much and underexercise make people fat. And these methods and beliefs form the foundation for eating disturbances. Think about it. If you are convinced that too much food and too little exercise make people fat, what are you going to do if you're worried about being thin enough? These theories must be abandoned if we're going to begin to make any real progress in rescuing people from the nightmare of food jail.

But why is the accepted treatment for obesity so important to consider in developing new prevention and treatment methods? Because it is our current approach to weight problems that dictates undereating as the way to stay thin, get thinner and lose weight to kids, young adults, everyone. Although undereating leads to weight loss, the rest of the story is never told. No one realizes what else undereating does to the body. People think it's benign. They believe that weight rebounding is about willpower or bad habits. They think dieting is good. The culture says it's right, healthy and necessary. All this has to change.

THE EMPOWERMENT OF THE NATURALLY THIN EATING PROGRAM

Naturally Thin eating is a program for preventing obesity and eating disorders, as well as for treating them. The Naturally Thin Program is a dramatic departure from the current treatment of these plagues because it is designed not to interfere with the body's natural urges, but to change the adaptive response pattern of the body in cooperation with the survival instinct. It does not assign superstitious causes to abnormal eating behavior because such behavior is understood as part of the adaptive response repertoire.

The theoretical framework of Naturally Thin—adaptation—offers practical methods for preventing adaptive weight gain, and implicates undereating as the culprit in both obesity and eating disturbances. Undereating, according to Naturally Thin, is not only not the solution for the weight conscious, it is the problem. And it is the problem for the eating disturbed as well.

With these insights, there is hope for the millions locked in food jail now, and for the inestimable numbers of kids who can be protected from eating disturbances in the future. But we are up against a Goliath in the $30 billion diet industry. Ours must be a quiet campaign of applying these principles to our own lives, teaching our kids, sharing with friends, reminding ourselves, insisting on change where we see the diet lie being told. Like Naturally Thin eating, there will be no dramatic, instant results. But over time, as we persist in telling the truth, the results will begin to show—in ourselves, our families, our schools, our communities, and eventually across the whole country. *Bon appétit!*

CHAPTER 9

When You Care About Someone Trapped in Food Jail

SO FAR WE HAVE FOCUSED OUR ATTENTION ON PEOPLE afflicted with eating disturbances, but they are not alone in their suffering. Although people with serious eating problems typically hide their symptoms, the lives of their families and other people close to them—friends and co-workers—are usually affected by their disorder, even if it is never discovered or acknowledged.

If you are the one with the eating problem, however successful you think you have been in hiding it, your struggle has impacted the people close to you. You may feel sure that no one knows, and you may be right. But even if you are, people who care about you have been affected by your eating troubles, no doubt about it. This isn't a guilt trip—it's about the reality of eating disturbances.

And to all the "concerned others" who are reading: you're not crazy, you're not responsible, and you can get through this, no matter what she (or he) decides to do.

• "I THOUGHT I WAS LOSING MY MIND"—*Natalie's Mom*

In the middle of a disappointing career change, Natalie's mom, a college professor, went to see a counselor. After a few sessions discussing the letdown and frustration of her job change, she began to talk at length about her troubled relationship with her daughter Natalie. She wasn't sure what the problem was, or even if there was one, whether it was Natalie or she who had the problem.

Natalie was a good student and very popular. At sixteen she had a boyfriend, but they didn't seem too serious. What

*worried her mother was a feeling that Natalie was hiding
something from her. Natalie seemed on edge quite a bit, and
her mother didn't think it could be hormones every day of the
month. Natalie was very moody, too. One day she'd be happy
and affectionate, making silly jokes—almost giddy—and the
next day she'd turn sad and depressed, hiding out in her
room whenever she was home. For a while Natalie's mom
thought it was just a teenage stage and let it go at that, but the
tension at home was getting worse, and she had started fighting with Natalie about her behavior.*

*When Natalie was down, the only response her mom got
from her was, "I'm fine. Leave me alone!" But when she was
in a good mood, Natalie laughed at her mother, "Mom, you're
paranoid. There's nothing wrong."*

*Natalie was so busy these days, her mom told the counselor,
that she never even had time to eat a meal at home. In fact,
when she was home, the only thing she took out of the refrigerator was diet pop. "Is she dieting?" the counselor asked.
"She's been dieting since she was thirteen," Natalie's mom
replied. "There's something wrong, something worse than dieting, or I really am going crazy."*

*Almost two years later Natalie admitted that she was bu-
limic and had been since she was fifteen.*

CONFUSING SYMPTOMS OF EATING DISORDERS

People with disturbed eating display quite an array of symptoms that can be confusing to those around them, especially if the
eating problem is a secret. But this long list of symptoms makes
sense when you understand that these troubled individuals are in
a serious fight with their bodies' instinct to survive. These symptoms reflect the body's and psyche's grave battle, and although
many physical symptoms are not evident to others, emotional and
behavioral symptoms often are.

Here's a list of the most common telltale symptoms of eating
disturbances:

1. anxiety, especially about food and eating
2. need for control over eating
3. secrecy, sneaking

4. mood swings, moodiness
5. depression
6. exaggerated sense of power to control/limit eating
7. preoccupation with food and eating
8. obsessiveness about food, weight, body shape
9. irrational thinking, behavior, especially regarding food and body size
10. irritability
11. guilt and shame
12. other symptoms associated with chronic hunger:
    weakness
    poor motivation
    trouble concentrating
13. excessive appetite
14. loss of control of eating behavior (bingeing)
15. loss of control of eating avoidance (self-starvation)
16. fear of loss of control over eating
17. distorted body image
18. perfectionism

These symptoms don't look the same in everyone. There are different combinations of symptoms, all in different degrees for each person who suffers from an eating problem. In the early stages, there may be few or no symptoms at all. Generally, the symptoms are milder for moderate dieters on the Feast or Famine Cycle and grow more serious as the degree of food avoidance increases.

It's easy to see, from this list, how people close to someone with such stressful and disturbing symptoms could become very upset themselves. And that's exactly what happens all too often. Caring people get sucked into a problem that they can't do much about, and it can make them sick, too. Let's take a look at what the pattern looks like and why this happens.

CO-DEPENDENCE AND EATING DISORDERS

Let's get more specific about how the symptoms of eating disorders affect the people close to the one who is sick. Any person's self-destructive behavior tends to pull those who care about her into a natural struggle. The urge to help, to rescue, to fix and to set right what is wrong is very powerful, especially in parents and spouses. We feel it's our job to save a person we love from danger and pain, and most of us will go to great lengths to try to do this.

This sounds noble, and it is so universal that it appears to be instinctive. But there are ways to "help" that aren't helpful at all, and even backfire, making the situation worse and the person sicker than before. When people try to help others they care about in unhelpful, self-defeating or even destructive ways, we call them co-dependent. Let me explain.

ASSESSMENT FOR CO-DEPENDENCE

Most people have some co-dependent tendencies. By "co-dependent" I mean "overconnected to a dependent, or unhealthy, person." And a person is dependent if she or he is trying to cope with life in self-destructive ways. People with eating disturbances are dependent, and people who are overconnected to them often try to cope with them and their problems in self-destructive ways. This is why we call them co-dependent.

> *Toni is a compulsive overeater, or bulimic. Her husband, Al, is so sympathetic to her struggle that he helps her search for a new diet whenever she gains weight, even calling the various companies and making appointments for her. He helps her count calories and fat grams. In fact, it's hard to tell just who is on the diet! And then, after Toni has successfully avoided all the bad foods and empty calories, and starved herself down to a lower weight, Al is right there with the goodies to reward her. He'll even run to the store in the middle of the night for her every craving. When Toni gains the weight back, Al is more depressed than she. This pattern has gone on for fourteen years.*

Here are the symptoms of co-dependence:

1. anxiety
2. need to control others
3. secrecy, sneaking
4. mood swings, moodiness
5. depression

6. exaggerated sense of power over others
7. preoccupation with dependent person
8. obsessiveness about dependent's problem
9. irrational thinking, behavior
10. irritability
11. exaggerated sense of responsibility
12. guilt and shame
13. poor personal boundaries (enmeshed with dependent person)
14. perfectionism

You probably thought you were reading the page on symptoms of eating disorders all over again. You weren't, but almost. The lists are remarkably similar because dependency tends to take on the same characteristics no matter what a person ends up dependent upon. The one with the so-called primary dependency looks just like the one who becomes secondarily dependent by getting overinvested in the dependent person. Most of their symptoms are identical, although they are usually provoked by different concerns.

Are you co-dependent? Have you developed some of these symptoms because of your relationship with the person in your life who has eating problems? First, look at the preceding list and circle the symptoms you have that are related to this concern. Then check your behavior and thinking for co-dependence:

True or False

1. ____ I worry about the person with an eating problem a lot.
2. ____ At times I can't concentrate because of my concern.
3. ____ I try to figure out ways to get through to her/him—to get her/him to admit she/he has a problem.
4. ____ I feel guilty, as if I'm to blame for the eating disturbance.
5. ____ I feel responsible to help her/him, no matter what.
6. ____ I don't think she/he can get well if I don't help.
7. ____ I believe that if I just work hard enough, I'll get through to her/him.
8. ____ I feel completely hopeless about this at times.
9. ____ This situation is getting to me emotionally.
10. ____ I lose my temper more since I found out about her/his eating problem.
11. ____ Sometimes I think I'm going crazy myself.

12.____I've spent a lot of time reading about eating disorders, looking for clues to understand her/him.

13.____I know I shouldn't spy, but I've secretly looked for evidence—hidden food, laxatives, diuretics, etc.

14.____There are times when I can't get this situation out of my mind.

15.____Sometimes I find myself saying or doing things I don't really want to, just to avoid conflict with this person.

NO PROBLEM HERE

Like most dependencies, eating disturbances are usually blanketed by a thick layer of denial. This defense, often shared by victim and "concerned persons" alike, is aided and abetted by the prevalence of dieting in our culture. Anyone who isn't dieting knows others who are. In fact, the nondieter seems, at this point, to be in the minority. Consequently, the eating disturbed are camouflaged. Their primary symptom—undereating—is not considered a symptom at all, but a sign of health and self-control. People with serious eating problems are difficult to identify, especially in the critical early stages, and coupled with their typical efforts to cover up their eating (or noneating) behavior, they can be securely locked up in food jail before anyone notices that something is wrong.

Denial is not a sin. And it isn't usually something people do on purpose. It is a valuable subconscious defense that keeps out information that threatens us. We need it and it serves us well at times. But denial can also keep a blindfold on our eyes when we desperately need to see what is before us.

Annie's mom was almost wild with worry. Her fifteen-year-old daughter had wasted down to skin and bones from a healthy, curvy shape only a year before. She had tried to talk to Annie many times, and was afraid she might be anorectic, but her biggest obstacle was her husband. He couldn't see what she did. When she shared her fears, he just said, "She's a teenager. They all do fad diets at this age. She'll be fine." His calm denial reassured Annie's mom that her daughter's weight and eating problems weren't worth getting hysterical over, and would probably go away by themselves if she were just patient. But her husband's denial of his daughter's symptoms delayed the intervention she desperately needed for over six months.

It helps to know what to look for if we are trying to face up to some suspicion about someone who may have an eating problem. Here are some general clues that may confirm or possibly refute your worry:

Common Behaviors and Clues Associated with Eating Disturbances

1. rigid eating behavior, refusal to eat regular foods
2. preoccupation with weight and dieting, frequent talk about food or losing weight
3. compulsive exercise, jogging in blizzards or during illness
4. eating very large amounts of food at one sitting, or eating nothing; immoderate eating
5. extreme pickiness about eating, eating only certain limited foods
6. frequent complaints that she is too fat when she is not
7. broken blood vessels in the eyes, dark circles around eyes
8. meal preparation for others but refusal to eat
9. expert knowledge of calorie and fat contents of many foods
10. prescription diuretics with no medical need
11. consistent time spent in bathroom following meals
12. denial of ever being hungry
13. complaints of hunger but refusal to eat
14. preoccupation with "fat" body part (e.g., complaints of "huge" thighs or bottom not consistent with reality.)
15. very frequent reading of diet books, nutrition books, cook books
16. stock of laxatives
17. stock of hidden food
18. eating in secret

WHERE DO YOU GO FROM HERE?

When you discover with certainty that someone you care about has an eating disturbance, first accept the fact. Don't let yourself rationalize away something you know is true simply because you don't want to believe it. Avoiding the reality of an eating problem because it's such an uncomfortable topic is a common reaction. But if you care enough to notice, to be sure, to face it, then stay with it.

If you are shaken by this awareness, perhaps because this is your wife or daughter or friend, you might consider seeing a counselor yourself before taking any other steps. You may need some reassurance that your suspicions are correct because if they aren't you may cause unnecessary conflict. Eating struggles are usually frightening, but a panicky approach will probably backfire. Take care of yourself first so you'll be better equipped to offer help to the one you love.

Next, make a decision about whether or not to confront the person. You don't have to, and depending on your relationship, it may not be appropriate. For example, your adult co-worker is obviously bulimic, but you don't have a close personal relationship, and her health seems OK otherwise. If you feel it's not appropriate to intervene, then just be aware of this problem in relating to her and try not to add to her struggle. For instance, be aware of her sensitivity concerning her weight, body, diet, etc. Be reassuring and supportive, but don't try to take care of her. You can't, and it won't help her—or you.

Of course, there are times when you must go further, even if you don't want to. These situations involve teens, or young adults away from home but still dependent, with symptoms at any level, or anyone who exhibits serious symptoms of eating disturbance: obvious physical or mental impairment including emaciation, fainting and suicide threat. If it appears that a person's life or safety may be in danger, it is your responsibility to act. You do not necessarily have to be the one who intervenes, but you must tell someone who will—a parent, teacher, husband, friend, pastor— anyone who cares and will follow through. In the case of a minor, the parents must be informed, too.

If you're the one to follow through, when you've settled down a bit, share your concern with a trusted friend who is more objective. Discuss different ways to handle your discovery, including an attempt to have a talk with this person. This is a rehearsal. It helps to minimize the surprises so you don't have to ad-lib too much when you do the real thing and your emotions are stretched.

If you decide to bring up the subject with a person close to you who has an eating disturbance, be prepared for denial, anger, accusations, threats, temper tantrums and possibly tears. These are common reactions when people with secret problems are found out, and it's not a pretty sight. They generally don't want to be found out, and they make that perfectly clear, one way or another, when you tell them you know.

You may not get an emotional tornado, but the point is, don't expect to hear, "Oh, thank goodness someone finally noticed! I really appreciate your concern. You are absolutely right—I have an eating disorder and I need help."

> Leah recalls: "I was furious when my mother started telling me to eat more. She called me anorectic. I said I hated her. I told her I couldn't live with her anymore—and I was only fourteen. I screamed at the top of my lungs, 'GET OUT OF MY LIFE—I CAN'T STAND THE SIGHT OF YOU.' I actually said all this to my own mother. She was just worried, but I didn't care. I couldn't bear the intrusion, the idea of anyone trying to interfere with my eating. I needed to do it my way, period."

Eating disturbances are supposed to be a secret. No one is supposed to realize that people close by (in their own house!) are completely fixated on food, bingeing, making themselves sick and starving their bodies, sometimes to death. This is why there is such a terrible reaction when the secret is discovered.

But why such a big secret? Why don't people with eating disorders just do their weird starving and bingeing out in the open? Because the very heart of eating disorders—control—would certainly be threatened if anyone found out, as Leah's mom did. Deep down these tortured souls seem to be aware that their eating patterns are so destructive that no one who found out would allow them to continue. And another thing: Disturbed eating behavior is shameful for many people. They know there's something wrong about it. They often feel so ashamed and embarrassed about their eating problems that they tell absolutely no one about their hidden life. So when they are discovered, victims of eating struggles are filled with two powerful and heavy emotions: fear of losing the control they fight so hard to maintain, and anger at having their shame uncovered.

There's one more reason for secrecy—denial. A person with an eating disorder may not be completely consciously aware of it. She may not be able to face it, so she denies it and keeps it hidden. When an outsider brings it up, there may be a violent reaction—a broken friendship, a move away from home, a letter of resignation. This reflects how serious the threat of the disclosure is, as well as the power of denial.

So now you know your sister or friend or daughter or wife has an eating disturbance. How can you possibly breach this subject with the likelihood of such a massive defense response? Deliberately—and carefully. In all fairness to eating-disturbed persons, it's never easy to hear someone, especially someone close to you, tell you that you're doing something wrong, no matter what that something is. But since this is a particularly charged topic, what is the best way to bring it up? What would be the most effective way to get the message through—that you care about this person, and that you know about her eating problem and want to help?

Remember the adage, "Give a compliment before you make a criticism"? I know it sounds simplistic and trite, but the idea has merit, and it applies here. Without getting syrupy or saccharine, first tell the person you care for why you want to have this talk—not about the eating problem, but about the person she is. Remind her that you care, just how much you value your relationship, that you love her and wouldn't want anything to ever happen to her. Mention some of the important things she brings into your life, her uniqueness, how she can't be replaced—those support messages reassuring her that she is much more than this problem you are about to bring up, and of course, she is.

Then say what you saw, the things you noticed (she will react to being spied upon) and why you think these things suggest to you that she may have some sort of eating problem. Do not accuse or use an accusing tone of voice. This is not a crime you are talking about, it is a type of sickness. Don't pretend you know all about her problem. Don't act as if you are a professional. Try to keep a "let's explore this together" atmosphere. If you can share what you learned from reading or seeing a counselor without pushing her away, then do that, but pay close attention to her responses. You'll know when you've said enough, and it might be right after your opening sentence!

> *"My best friend was the first one to suspect anything," Rebecca remembers. "She knew I'd tried throwing up so I wouldn't gain weight—she had tried it, too. But when she was sure I was stuck [on the Cycle], she just told me how worried*

she was and asked me if I was worried, too. I was. She stayed on my side when she brought it up and told me she understood my fears about getting fat. She didn't try to argue with me—that was important. Even though I basically denied everything that first time we talked about it, when I was ready, she became my biggest support when I was getting off the Cycle. I don't think I could have done it without her."

It's important to distinguish between a chronic/stable eating disorder and an acute/dangerous one when deciding how far you should go in an intervention. You might be able to help or support the person with the former type by giving her information about the Cycles because she is not in physical danger. But people in the acute/dangerous stages need professional help, and if you try to help them yourself, they might not get it.

CHRONIC/STABLE EATING DISORDERS

Chronic/stable eating disorders are in no way benign, but they usually do not involve medical emergencies. These include the Feast or Famine Cycle disturbances of compulsive overeating, food addiction and chronic yo-yo dieting, and disturbances brought on by Cycle variations, including all of these plus infrequent purging with drugs, exercise or vomiting (mild bulimia).

In order to qualify as chronic and stable, a person's weight range must be near normal or above. Undereating and overeating, even with occasional purging by vomiting, exercise or laxative abuse, can usually be tolerated over many years. And they are, by millions of people, many of whom are never identified as eating disturbed. The eating patterns they grow accustomed to almost become normal for them. These people do not need an intervention per se, nor do they require medical help. But their eating problems, although well tolerated physically, are almost never easy on the emotions or self-esteem. They do need the information in this book. Without it they are likely to stay locked in food jail indefinitely.

ACUTE/DANGEROUS EATING DISORDERS

Acute/dangerous eating disorders are different. They are certainly health-threatening and sometimes life-threatening as well. Watch for:

Feast or Famine Cycling (see page 60) that is extreme: diets that require fasting, all liquid diets, very low calorie diets (under 1,000 calories), very rapid weight loss, very rapid rebound weight gain, severe calorie restriction (under 1,200 calories) with vigorous exercise, weight loss 10 percent below normal, serious depression.

FeaFam Cycling (see page 71) that is acute/dangerous: bulimia when purging follows most or all eating episodes, daily or very regular abuse of laxatives and/or diuretics, inability to keep food down (reflex vomiting), weight loss 10 percent below normal, serious depression.

Famine Track (see page 75) or anorectic eating with these symptoms: weight loss 10 percent below normal, refusal to eat at all, eating only miniscule amounts, very restrictive diet with vigorous exercise, fainting, dizziness, absence of menstrual periods, social isolation, an alarming gaunt or sickly appearance, serious weight loss that accompanies drug abuse, drug dependency, depression.

The acute/dangerous eating disorder symptoms cannot be ignored because they reflect at least a potentially serious physical threat. And naturally, if you are close to someone and you recognize earlier symptoms of these dangerous disorders, you'll want to intervene sooner. A lot depends on your relationship.

Parents of minor children have the most power to influence a child in the early stages of an eating disturbance. They don't have to have the cooperation of the kid to get her/him to professional help. Not so with just about everybody else. Fortunately, perhaps, these disorders most often get started during early adolescence, when they are easier to detect because parents are around to observe, and the child eats at home, at least some of the time. (We'll explore this more fully in Chapter 10: Keeping Kids Out of Food Jail.)

GETTING OUTSIDE HELP

If the eating disturbance is acute/dangerous, the best thing to do is to get professional help. Just getting the person to a doctor for a physical should be the goal in this situation because the physical threat is paramount. Any physician, including the family doctor, will do. You should be referred to a specialist if it's necessary. The only exception to this is a situation where there is a potential for suicide. Then you should try to see a psychiatrist. Find one who specializes in eating disorders, if possible.

It's impossible to tell how serious the sick person's condition is unless she is examined and has lab tests run. Don't project into the future with the person you are trying to help, talking about treatment or therapy. She doesn't need a barrage of "threats" at this point. Just stick with the physical as the goal. When the results are in, the doctor will help her (and you, if you are the parent and she is a minor) decide what the next step should be. If you are not related or this relative is an adult, this may be the end of your helping role.

If the person you love is referred to an eating disorders program and you are a family member, there will probably be some help offered for you. And if you are not a family member, you may be able to participate as a concerned friend. Now it's time for you to get help for yourself and take the focus off the person you have brought.

Steering Away from Co-Dependence: Guidelines to help you be more effective in helping those you love

Here are some simple rules to follow to help you make decisions about helping the person you care about. It's a good idea to check any idea against this list before deciding on any action you think would be helpful. If your idea conforms to these guidelines, then go ahead. If not, better hold off.

1. Take Good Care of Yourself. Stay in touch with your own needs and limitations. If you have considerable trouble with this, see a counselor yourself. You can probably use the support anyway.

2. Don't Get in Over Your Head. Don't try to be an eating disorders counselor. If you feel that the situation is dangerous, or potentially so, get professional advice. If the person with an eating disturbance won't go for professional help, find out what you should do, and get some support for yourself.

3. Stay Focused on Your Own Life. It's easy to get sucked into the worry world of crazy eating. Don't do it. Do not allow yourself to obsess about the sick person—it will drain you, and it won't help her. Schedule projects or activities you enjoy for your free time if you are unable to keep your mind off the situation. And if you simply can't keep your thoughts in line, see a counselor.

4. Tell the Secret. Besides the professional avenues of support, it's helpful if you tell someone close to you, whom you trust, about the problem. Tell more than one person if you can, so you have options when you need to talk. Do not keep this a secret, no matter how ashamed you may feel about it. You shouldn't be in this alone.

5. Back Off Emotionally from the Sick Person. This doesn't mean abandonment. It means taking a mental step back from a person who can too easily "hook" your emotions in an unhealthy way. It's also called detachment, and it's a method for setting better boundaries between you and the person you care about. Practicing "seeing" the person as a stranger or acquaintance may help you achieve detachment.

6. Back Off Physically, Too. This doesn't mean that you should stop showing affection, it's about respecting the personal space and the physical lines between people. For example, avoid watching the person who worries you choose food or eat. Leave the room if necessary. Make no comments about what you see regarding her choices. Do not go through her personal belongings, looking for "evidence." You may not like what you find, and if you don't find anything you'll still be worried.

7. Limit Sharing Your Concerns. It's senseless to try to hide your worries from a confidant. So after you've brought the subject up once, and found professional help if the person is in danger, limit the times (i.e., once a week) that you share your continued concern. This is called containing your feelings and it is different from suppressing them, only to have them come out later. Talking about them at specific times will help

you contain them at others, or deal with them with the support of other people.

8. Practice "Tough Love." When we love someone it's natural to try to protect them from pain. But the pain that comes from eating problems may be the only motivator for the suffering person to change or get help. So don't interfere with that pain. Don't cover up for her, don't make it easier for her to hide, to believe this is normal, to manage her bizarre lifestyle. This is a big challenge, but it is extremely important.

Molly and Katherine were first cousins sharing a small apartment on a college campus. They got along well and shared most responsibilities of apartment living, including grocery shopping. Their first major crisis happened shortly after Molly realized that something was wrong with Katherine's eating. Until that time each took a turn grocery shopping for the week and the other one made a list of things she wanted. As Katherine's list became more and more "unusual," Molly felt she had to say something.

"I can't buy this stuff for you, Kate, it's all rabbit food. You're thin as a rail. You're not eating enough," Molly declared.

"Just because I eat healthy food and you eat junk doesn't mean the problem is mine," Katherine countered. "You agreed to shop every other week, so you have to. Besides, it's none of your business what I eat. Everybody's thin compared to you."

That last crack really hurt, even though Molly wasn't overweight. Molly's voice was shaking as she responded, "It is my business if you're killing yourself. I think you're getting anorectic and I don't want to see you get sicker. I won't buy your so-called health food. You get your groceries, I'll get mine. I wish you'd get help."

Katherine didn't get help, but Molly stuck to her decision.

Tough love is not about manipulating someone into doing what we want them to. It's about letting another person know that her lifestyle, and its consequences, is what it really is, without artificial softeners. By the way, your refusal to cooperate with someone's self-destructive habits will probably incite anger and possibly rage. These emotions are meant to keep you in line, force you, from fear of the reaction you'll get, to do whatever the dependent person wants: keep quiet, buy supplies, support delusions, play dumb, etc.

SOME INEFFECTIVE THINGS CONCERNED PEOPLE DO WHEN THEY'RE WORRIED AND/OR CONFUSED

When caring people become alarmed about some danger to a person they love, particularly when it is self-inflicted, they often react with tactics that are designed to help them feel in better control of the situation. This happens especially when the people who are reacting clearly have little or no control over the situation. Naturally, the discovery of pathological eating in a loved one usually fits this pattern. It often evokes panicky attempts to get some sort of foothold on the problem, or a foothold on the person with the problem.

Taking Control

The most obvious way a "concerned other" tries to fix the pain he feels about someone's eating problem is by trying to control that someone. "There's not going to be any bulimia in my house," a frightened father shouts at his wife when he learns of his nineteen-year-old's purging. "I'll follow her around after she eats so she won't be able to throw up. I'll check her purse and packages for laxatives. You'll see how long she can keep this up while I'm around." It's his fear, and perhaps his shame, that inspires such unrealistic vows. But behind the fear and shame is his love for his daughter. He does not know what to do, and his helplessness is intolerable to him.

Advice-Giving

Well-meaning friends and relatives, when faced with the upsetting news of an eating disturbance in someone they love, sometimes cope with their concern by playing the expert. The mother of a newly diagnosed anorectic shares the news with her sister, the girl's aunt. This is her response: "Well, you remember Aunt Harriet, don't you? She had a touch of anorexia, too, and they sent her on a trip to fatten her up, to Florida. It worked, too. They said it was her depression that made her so thin. But she got over it.

You should send Beth on a trip. She just needs a change of scenery. Let me talk to her. We'll get this straightened out." You can hear the subtle fear in her comments, just beneath a veneer of confidence. Most people don't know how to say, or aren't comfortable saying, "I'm sorry to hear that, and I'm afraid because I know that anorexia can be very serious."

Lecturing

Parents are especially prone to this response when their anxiety is triggered. In fact, children grow so accustomed to it that they can predict which lecture is likely to accompany certain situations. "When my mom found out I was throwing up my food, she lectured me straight for over an hour," Deirdre remembers. "I think she brought in every major point she had ever used before, she was so upset. I heard all these, and more: 'how much your dad and I love you' and 'how could you let us down after all we've done for you' and 'on top of all I have to cope with, now I have this to worry about.' I felt a little guilty, like I was a burden to her, but her speech didn't affect my eating. That was my business."

Threats

When an eating disorder is discovered, sometimes concerned persons use threats to conquer their fear of the unknown, to force the sick person into straightening out or else.

Ashley was furious when she accidentally stumbled on her sister's drawer of purge aids—boxes of laxatives, a bottle of prescription diuretics and even a bottle of syrup of ipecac (normally used to induce vomiting in poison victims). Her anger was obvious when she immediately confronted her sister, who made excuses and denied that she had a problem. This upset Ashley even more. "Do you know what you're doing to yourself? You're going to die if you keep this up. Your body will never be normal. You'll never be able to have children. I know someone who ended up in a mental hospital because she did this stuff so long. I won't let you do this. If you keep this up, I won't be around to watch you destroy yourself. You're going to be all alone."

Guilt-Tripping

Guilt is a potent motivator in some susceptible individuals, but it is inappropriate for getting through to people with troubled eating patterns. This is because their rigid priorities usually don't allow guilt, however real, to interfere significantly with their eating. Then the guilt only damages the relationship and/or the person's self-worth.

> *Alyssa's mom was visibly upset as she described the struggle with her daughter to a counselor: "Each time I told Alyssa how much it hurt me to see her starving herself, she seemed to eat even less. I didn't understand why she would try to hurt me even more." The counselor asked Alyssa about it and she explained: "Mom's guilting me really only made me mad. She had no right to interfere with my eating! It just intensified my determination to eat even less. It was how I got back at her for trying to make me feel guilty when my eating had nothing to do with her." Guilt-tripping often backfires.*

Manipulation and Bribes

Although these tactics are the cornerstones of eating disorders treatment when weight gain is paramount, they are usually ineffective in the long run when used in other situations. If privileges are withheld in order to motivate eating, or keep a person from purging behaviors, they usually have little or no lasting effect because the privileges earned don't amount to much when compared to the goal of The Thin Ideal.

> *Rhonda, diagnosed with anorexia when she was sixteen, shares her perspective: "Dad told me I couldn't drive the car until my weight was up ten pounds. That was a year ago. I just don't drive anymore. He's offered me money, too, but he just doesn't get it. I can't gain weight for anything."*
>
> *Rhonda reflects the power of the food trap—the threatening adapted appetite and the necessity of maintaining rigid controls over eating, in spite of significant losses. A ten-pound gain is a terrifying impossibility to someone caught on the Famine Track. Bribes and manipulations are clearly impotent to set these people free.*

Shame

A common and desperate response to frightening information about a person we love is shame. It's a paradox that our love takes this form at times, but fear, as we have seen, takes many forms in distorting the message of love. Shame is a deep sense of inadequacy, of defectiveness. It's different from guilt because it isn't associated with our behavior, it's about our personhood. When we experience shame, we feel unworthy and insecure. When we shame someone, we attack her basic sense of self at the core. Such deep wounds are most often inflicted by people who love each other.

The shame repertoire is large, but here's a sampling of common shaming messages: "What's the matter with you? You're really sick, you know that? Why can't you eat like a normal human being? You're disgusting. I can't stand the sight of you. Can't you do anything right? Do you always have to invent new ways to make me sick? Why can't you be like your sister? You're never going to be able to accomplish anything as long as you eat like this, that's for sure."

Shame is a way of pulling the psychological rug out from under someone. It is powerful, and that's why people who love people who are in trouble use it. It's supposed to make the person in danger feel so terrible about herself that she will decide to change her self-destructive behavior. Although shame usually does plenty of damage, it doesn't get people to change seriously for the better.

Rejection

Sally, who lived with her aunt and uncle off campus while she attended a private high school, explained how this tactic affected her: "My aunt and uncle found out about my bingeing from my counselor at school. They had been suspicious, but when someone else told them they totally hit the roof and called me everything from a neurotic to a slob. I was really overweight, but that didn't seem to be such a big deal until they found out I was bingeing big time. Then they told me I couldn't live with them anymore, that I'd have to live in the dorm, which they knew I couldn't afford. They actually threw me out because of my eating problem. I think they thought I'd 'snap out of it' if they completely rejected me. But I couldn't

snap out of it, and our relationship was almost destroyed by
their reaction."

Another young bulimic describes how his peers reacted to
learning about his eating disorder. "When they found out about it,
you'd think I had the plague. I was ostracized. I could feel their rejection from across a room. It got so bad that I finally changed
schools. I was careful to keep it a secret at the new school."

Abuse

People who are worried about someone they love use control,
give advice, lecture, threaten, guilt-trip, manipulate, bribe, shame
and reject in order to feel better themselves. All these tactics are
abusive—attempts to fix their heavy feelings—and instead of helping anyone, these methods often end up hurting the person they
are worried about. Remember, people with eating disturbances
are already in a fair amount of pain, just struggling with their
symptoms, which include deep fear, shame and confusion. They
don't need to be emotionally beaten into facing their disorder;
they need to be educated into facing it, without manipulation,
psychological pressures or cruelty.

PROFESSIONAL HELP—PROS AND CONS

On the plus side of seeking professional help for eating problems is the reassurance of people who are familiar with these disturbances. Eating struggles seem so foreign to most people, and
are consequently quite frightening. It is very helpful, indeed, just
to hear a counselor respond to the list of symptoms we share with
a knowing, "Yes, that's common." Somehow, just the word "common" feels better to us, no matter how bizarre the behavior we
have described. When we feel helpless, just to be able to reach out
to someone wiser, stronger and more capable than ourselves is a
primitive need. So it's valuable that professionals in this field play
the role of the reassuring and wise helper.

There is another aspect of professional help for eating problems
offered today that has merit. It is nutritional counseling. But even
these benefits are limited in many cases because the real incentive
to eat more food and stop going hungry—to break out of food

jail—is never really presented. The reasons that are given—to be healthier, to get your period back, to get your parents off your back, etc.—are often not enough when held up against the paramount reason to continue undereating: weight control. This applies to anorectics and bulimarectics who, professionals acknowledge, have an undereating problem, although it is usually considered secondary to psychological factors.

Nutritional counseling for anorectics is usually well attended because anorectics would rather talk about food and nutrition than anything else. But talking about nutrition and eating is one thing, and actually learning why and how to eat more food is another. This is where the nutritional advice is limited, but it is still the most valuable aspect of treatment happening today. Unfortunately, it is never the focal point of treatment.

Bulimics are not seen by professionals in general as undereaters. Food addicts and compulsive overeaters aren't either. The focal symptom of these bulimic groups is binge eating. And the focus of treatment is not nutritional advice but finding the psychological reasons for the bingeing and purging. Much is made of binge/purge behavior, as professionals log feelings and experiences connected to these behaviors, but they almost never address the question of why bulimics need to binge and how eating more prevents bingeing. Again, the importance of increasing overall food intake is ignored, and consequently, bulimics continue to undereat. As long as they do, they binge and purge, too. It's food jail.

In a capsule, modern therapies for eating disorders almost completely ignore the central role of undereating in these disorders because they have historically been considered psychological illnesses. There is so much presumption of psychological factors that at times it looks ridiculous.

Gen attended a famous clinic for anorexia where part of her therapy consisted of watching a movie and then visiting with a therapist afterward to discuss the feelings that she had during the movie. "It was stupid," she recalls. "I did it because it was the only way to get out of there, but it was like they thought if I just get my feelings out, I'd start eating. But I wasn't going to start eating for all the feelings in the world. The reason is simple: if I ate more I'd gain weight."

So-called food addicts are sometimes treated in clinics for ad-dictions. Their undereating is usually ignored, especially since they are almost always overweight. And compulsive overeaters are never, as their label implies, taken to be undereaters. If they were, the professionals ask, how could they be so fat? The nutritional counseling these groups receive often includes low-fat, calorie-re-stricted diets. If these diets are followed (and often they aren't be-cause they are considered "too much food"), they only promote the Cycle that causes the symptoms for which the person sought help in the first place.

What to Look For When You Get Help

With these limitations in mind, when you seek help for some-one who has an eating disturbance, or for yourself, here's a check-list to help you gather helpful information. A physician or psychiatrist should be involved if the disorder is acute/dangerous.

1. Check out the clinics, hospital programs and individual thera-pists available. (Some of you may not have much to choose from.) Make a list of your options.
2. Write down all the things you want from the program or ther-apist.
3. Find out how much nutritional counseling is available.
4. Find out what the central focus of therapy will be. If under-eating is ignored, keep looking.
5. Often family therapy is helpful because it gives people a chance to air their feelings, so find out if that's a possibility.
6. With the person who needs help, meet the therapist or dietit-ian who will be in charge, to assess the personality match. If you don't get a good feeling, ask to switch to another.
7. If you don't want psychotherapy, try to find a dietitian who works with clients with disturbed eating.
8. If you want someone who will integrate the Naturally Thin principles into therapy, take this book and ask. Dietitians are your best bet.
9. Keep taking care of yourself. If the person who concerns you refuses to accept the help you offer, and you have no lever-age (she lives on her own and is an adult), it's time to let go.

LETTING GO

When people we love are determined to live in a way that is dangerous and potentially lethal, it goes against our emotional grain to let go of them, even when they push us away again and again. We want to hang on, to fight for them, against them, with them against the danger. But, as most parents, spouses, sisters, brothers and friends who have lost a long battle like this know, the sooner you let go and give responsibility for bearing the pain and solving the problem to the one with the problem, the better the odds that she/he'll come through it all right.

Why? A person with an eating problem is part of a system, or group of concerned people, and other members of that system are affected by her illness. These others can be so affected that they become sick, too, or co-dependent. Co-dependents tend to over-adjust to other people's problems so that the pain and disturbance of those problems is minimized. The person with the primary problem is cushioned by the co-dependent's overadjustments from the consequences of her/his self-destructive behavior. Put more simply, self-destructive lifestyles can be made relatively pain-free with the help of loyal co-dependents. This is more serious than it appears.

Co-dependents believe that their efforts to help the sick person are essential. Their lives tend to become focused on this "helping" role, sometimes to the exclusion of their own responsibilities. So convinced are they that their role is vital that they fail to see how destructive their behavior becomes. At best, they distract the sick person from the reality and danger of her/his illness, and at worst they make that sickness seem like a reasonable way to live. All this helps people get comfortable in food jail.

Letting go of a person with an eating disturbance means admitting that you can't do it for another person. It means respecting another person's choices, whether good or bad. It means getting down out of the control tower and on to a level playing field, where each person has his own struggle and must face his own troubles. It means allowing pain and frustration in another person's life because pain and frustration are normal parts of life that often cause growth. Letting go means releasing another to learn from her own experiences, however distressing they may be. And letting go is about giving up a belief in your power over another person. We are connected by systems, but we are separated, too, by our individuality.

Clearly, letting go is no picnic. But it's something even the sickest co-dependents can learn to do when they find out that they must, in order to really help the person they love.

WHEN YOU UNDERSTAND BUT THEY DON'T

In my work with families of people with eating problems, a situation often comes up that causes distress for concerned others who know about the physical component of eating disturbances, but the person or family they are worried about doesn't. Perhaps professional help has been sought, but because of the psychological focus and absence of information about the undereating key, there is no progress. This can be a problem if the relationship isn't strong, with a lot of trust. Whatever the relationship, it usually works out better if the ideas about the physical basis of eating disorders are shared briefly and then this book is offered. Even if the trapped person doesn't seem interested, sometimes she is open and will read about the Naturally Thin approach.

> Tricia had been "addicted to food," especially sweets, for most of her thirty-three years. She had just regained over forty pounds that had come off grudgingly with a very strict diet. She was very depressed about her weight gain and about the old, sick eating pattern that seemed to have possessed her again. She simply couldn't stay away from anything sweet, and she didn't have any hope of successfully dieting again.
>
> One discouraged Saturday morning, Tricia was surprised to find a package from her sister Rita in Canada. It was a book about the physical component of eating problems. Tricia wasn't aware that her sister even knew about her eating problems! She read the note: "You're not eating enough! Love, Rita." Tricia could only think, If you only knew!
>
> She read the first chapters, though without much hope, because she thought Rita would call and ask her what she thought about the book. Somewhere in Chapter 3, it clicked. Tricia began to understand what she had been doing to herself all these years, with her diets and starvation kicks, skipping meals and eating nearly nothing at others. Insight about

her undereating and her huge hunger for sweets hit her in a single moment. Big tears rolled down her cheeks. She was almost embarrassed by them even though she was alone. "I've never cried from reading a book!" she whispered to herself. But the tears kept coming.

Two weeks later Tricia called Rita. She was so excited that she could hardly wait for her sister to pick up the phone. "Rita, Rita, you won't believe it. I think I'm cured! I passed up candy and cookies today at a luncheon. I didn't want them. Do you believe it? I really didn't want to eat sweets. I'm so happy. Thank you, thank you, thank you for the book. I finally understand how this whole thing got started . . . and why it kept going. Thank you."

Tricia was ready for the information she received. Rita had no way of knowing that, but she did know about her sister's undereating—from her weight problem. She took a chance and it paid off, the same way it had helped her daughter overcome bulimarexia.

Struggling to stay off the Feast or Famine Cycle, Tricia spent almost four years getting down to the weight at which she felt comfortable. "It was a big switch for me, going from trying not to eat to trying to avoid going hungry, but I just took all the willpower I had used over the years to diet to learn to eat right," she recalls.

In the end, the most effective way you can help anyone caught in food jail is to show her the way she can really be set free. Without this information, her chances of breaking out are limited at best. With it, she can be truly liberated. But remember, when and whether she breaks out of food jail is ultimately up to her.

CHAPTER 10

Keeping Kids
Out of Food Jail

THE AMERICAN CANCER SOCIETY RECOMMENDATIONS for preventing cancer include this admonition: Avoid obesity. As if we weren't trying. And the way we're trying to avoid obesity is the same as it was forty years ago when pioneer researchers concluded that more than 95 percent of dieters regain all the weight they lose by dieting: We're still dieting. We're trying to eat less and exercise more.

It has been demonstrated conclusively for forty years that these behaviors do not lead to lasting leanness, and they do, unfortunately, lead many to disturbed eating patterns, increasing obesity and potentially damaging weight fluctuations. Recently, scientists in this field have expressed confusion over the ever-rising rates of obesity and eating disorders in this country, where dieting and dietary education, low-fat eating and physical fitness are only escalating in importance. We are still barking up the wrong tree when it comes to food problems, with serious and even grave consequences to many.

Effective eating-disturbance prevention requires changing trees. This means identifying and educating our children about the real culprits in obesity and eating disturbances: undereating, late eating and poor-quality eating; and especially the serious dangers of food-restricted dieting.

Three factors combine to produce eating disturbances in kids. The first is the powerful Thin Ideal message of the culture, without which eating disturbances are rather rare. So just being American puts kids at risk. The second factor is the child's own predisposi-

tion, including physical and personal qualities that prevent or enhance the development of eating problems. A child's sex comes in
here. A much higher percentage of girls than boys develop troubled eating. And the third influence is the social and familial environment of the young person.

Some of these characteristics have been associated with eating
disorders by professionals, and others I have observed in my own
work. Keep in mind that some, but usually not all, of these personality traits are found in young people with eating problems.

Kids at Risk: Personal Characteristics That Predispose a Child to Eating Disorders

1. adolescence
2. extreme focus on weight and appearance
3. emphasis on performance
4. strong will and determination
5. athlete/model/performer
6. high activity level, busy schedule
7. ability to block or dissociate from pain to achieve goal
8. black/white, all or nothing thinking
9. depression
10. perfectionism
11. high tolerance for hunger
12. female

The other ingredients that contribute to eating disorders come
from the child's environment, including her/his family.

Thirteen Ways Parents (and Other People Who Are Close to the Child) Can Encourage Eating Disorders

1. Be sure you yourself diet, and discuss your progress and
   problems in front of the child often.
2. Make a lot of disparaging remarks about your own weight
   and body size.
3. Always make cruel comments about overweight people you
   see in public.
4. Bring attention to her "chubby little body" from the time
   she is two or three. These are all made in fun, of course.
   (Naturally, it isn't necessary that she actually be chubby.)

5. Give her a nickname that reflects that "chubby little body," like Tubs or Donut.
6. Never affirm, compliment or encourage her about the appearance or shape of her body as it develops during childhood or adolescence.
7. Ignore her first attempts to diet or, better still, encourage dieting.
8. Really go crazy with praise and attention when she does lose weight by dieting.
9. If she gains the weight she lost back, frown and criticize her. Be sure to use her old nickname.
10. Keep sweets, junk food and dessert foods around the kid at all times, and not much else.
11. If she ever gets too thin, enthusiastically tell her to pursue a modeling career and take her shopping for a smaller-size wardrobe.
12. If she gains and actually becomes overweight, compare her to people in the family or neighborhood who are seriously overweight, warning her that she'll end up like that if she isn't careful.
13. When the eating disorder is finally diagnosed, look at her with abhorrence and exclaim, "How could you do this to me?"

DISCLAIMER FOR PARENTS

Does this list imply that parents, by their example and interactions with their children, single-handedly put them in food jail? No. Although we know that willful undereating for weight loss is the starting point for most eating disorders, apparently no single factor accounts for when and exactly why some particular kids start limiting their food intake in the first place. All we do know is that, with rare exception, the one common goal these kids have is weight loss.

The point of the list is this: Important people in a kid's life can heighten or minimize a child's inclination toward eating problems. If you found things on the list that you have done, take yourself off the hook right now. You were ignorant, you couldn't have known what you know now, you would have done it differently if you had known. Besides, you can't overlook the other influences, including your child's personality and talents, that powerfully impact kids' eating behavior today.

A most unfortunate reality for parents of kids with eating trouble is that they don't know what they might have done to prevent their kid from getting into food jail in the first place. Perhaps they themselves are caught in food jail. How can you warn your child about something if you don't even know how it happens or what to do to prevent it? And how can you explain it if you don't understand it yourself?

MISUNDERSTANDING OBESITY

As long as we believe that eating too much food by itself causes weight gain and obesity, we are doomed to send a message to our kids that will lead some of them into disturbed eating behaviors. And as long as we continue to allow the fashion and advertising industries to promote only the superthin standard especially for our daughters' bodies, we are bound to see more and more adolescent girls striving to achieve such bodies and the ever-increasing eating problems that result. And if we don't begin to see traditional dieting for what it really is—a damaging and dangerous method for weight loss which does not work and often backfires, causing weight gain—we are doomed to suffer increasing weight control and eating problems. These patterns and prejudices, along with their consequences, are already very much upon us.

EDUCATION VS. INDOCTRINATION

The very best defense against anything, they say, is education. But I have found that indoctrination works even better than that. For example, it's one thing to have a health teacher at school tell your kids that it's important for them to stay away from dieting and always eat good food when they get hungry. She might even explain the reasons behind her admonitions, talking about adaptation and how the body works to store fat in a famine environment. And she would certainly caution her students to be alert for the symptoms of the Feast or Famine Cycle, the starting point for all eating problems. Perhaps these health classes would touch on this subject once a year, and then, only after the curriculum is changed. This is education.

Indoctrination is something else altogether. A young mother starts by feeding her new babies on demand, and as they grow, she never changes her basic approach. As toddlers, preschoolers, school-age children, teenagers and young adults she feeds them on demand, just as she and her husband eat on demand.

"On demand" simply means that food is always available for hungry kids, period. Now, maybe the food available an hour before supper isn't meal-type food because the meal is coming up soon, but it is something decent, like fruit or cereal. Moms and dads who are indoctrinating their kids this way have some order, some meals eaten together, even though individual hunger signals govern eating behavior. There are patterns of hunger that permit regular meals to be scheduled without causing problems.

The first, and most important, part of indoctrination is:

> *Teach your kids to always eat on demand by always feeding them whenever they are hungry.*

Next, tell your kids how important it is that they listen to their bodies' hunger signals. This is completely natural for young children, but as they get older many kids get distracted by play or work and ignore hunger signals. Make their hunger a priority by responding to it appropriately, taking some action to help them get some good food. Ask them if they are hungry when you know it's been a few hours since they last ate. When they are older, tell them why it's important to never ignore their hunger. Nine-year-olds understand the principles of adaptation, and this insight can motivate them to eat well.

> *Teach your kids to listen to their own bodies.*

If you want your children to eat good food and avoid lousy food, keep plenty of good food around and don't buy lousy food. You don't have to be a nutritionist to figure which is which. Good foods are lower-fat meal-type foods and lousy foods are typically found in vending machines. They're also called snacks. Snack foods are entirely unnecessary and usually quite expensive. No one needs them. Kids do well eating sandwiches, cereal, fruit, breads, pizza and leftovers for snacks, between major mealtimes.

Make only good-quality Real Foods available to your kids.

Teach your kids from early on that dieting and trying to eat less than they want is unhealthy and leads to weight and appetite problems and eating disorders. Tell them that dieting is stupid. Have a "down with dieting" attitude. Don't diet and don't glamorize anyone who is dieting "successfully."

Encourage a negative attitude toward dieting.

Help your kids feel happy about their bodies by enjoying their unique physiques. Tell them they have good shapes, pleasing curves, strong muscles. Be alert to self-consciousness about a physical feature and reassure them of their attractiveness and their uniqueness. Support and reassure the ones who suffer from body-image crises when they compare themselves to more perfectly shaped peers. Emphasize their specialness, even including aspects of their bodies that they may not like. Keep in mind that adolescents are extremely concerned with their appearance, and almost all can benefit from warm acceptance of their physical selves at home.

Help your kids like their bodies.

It's a well-known fact that naturally thin people get their cues to eat from inside their bodies, from hunger signals. And most people with eating disturbances and weight problems get their cues to eat from outside themselves, from the clock or other people. Most little children don't question their hunger signals, but naturally seek food when they are hungry and eat until they are satisfied. If this pattern was never interfered with, we'd have a lot fewer eating troubles to worry about. Remind your kids that they can always trust the hunger signals their bodies send.

Teach your kids to trust their body signals.

Children learn from all around that overweight people got that way by eating too much all the time. Researchers have conceded during the last decade that the problem is much more complex than that. Obesity is a disorder of adaptation. Overweight represents an adaptive response to an environment where high-quality food is intermittently restricted. Overweight people are not eating enough good food some of the time, and that's what sets the whole adaptive response pattern in motion. Undereating, eating late—long after hunger is first felt—eating poor-quality food, skipping meals, ignoring hunger are the triggers for obesity and eating disorders.

Teach your kids that going hungry can cause weight gain and eating problems.

Your kids need to know the basic response that bodies have to undereating—the symptoms of the Feast or Famine Cycle. They need to know because some of them are going to Cycle as a result of their reckless eating, busy schedules, high activity level or attempts to lose weight. An awareness of these symptoms can give them the insight they'll need to change their eating patterns before they are locked in food jail.

The symptoms of the Feast or Famine Cycle, which parallel the body's adaptive response to famining, include: excessive hunger, a tendency to overeat or binge, cravings for sweets and/or fatty foods, the urge to eat without real hunger (especially at night), eating in response to stress or emotional upset, special occasion overeating and preoccupation with food.

Make your kids familiar with the symptoms of the Feast or Famine Cycle.

If you have a weight or eating problem, don't drag your kid into the struggle. You can seek support from plenty of other people. Demonstrate, instead, an appreciation of your own body, with all its imperfections and limitations. And take care of your body. Eat well yourself. Don't go hungry. Don't eat junk. Get some exercise every day or two. Wear attractive clothes that fit. Don't let your physical liabilities cramp your style, and your kid isn't likely to either.

Accept your own body with grace.

Be alert to the cultural standard for thinness that your kids are exposed to every day. Don't support this standard and be vocal about your attitude. Let your kids know that the fashion pictures and advertisements in their magazines aren't realistic standards for healthy adolescents. For example, you might point out the ridiculously gaunt arms and legs of a model advertising cigarettes. Never compare your kids to these standards in ways that tell them their bodies aren't the way they should be. And be prepared to cushion and debate a mean remark about your kid's body or weight made by peers or even a teacher or coach.

Remind your kids that The Thin Ideal is not ideal or even normal for most people.

If you follow these recommendations, are your kids completely immune from developing disturbed eating? No, they aren't. But they are much less likely to be locked in food jail than kids who are left wide open to the pervasive messages of the culture: food is bad and thin is perfect.

UNDERSTANDING WEIGHT GAIN

In order to discourage the dieting that sets kids up for food jail, we have to teach them about the Feast or Famine Cycle—why weight gain is adaptive when people go hungry or eat too-low-quality food. Kids must grasp the reality of how adaptive weight gain happens and learn that the true underlying cause of weight gain is undereating good food. Since the central task of dieting is undereating, dieting would naturally be avoided by many kids who understand these principles. If kids get the message that going hungry sets them up to gain weight, they are more likely to eat when they should—when they are hungry—and eat better food. And if they are better fed, their appetites will be more manageable, and they will be much less likely to eat low-class food out of desperation.

Once kids understand that undereating will never lead to permanent weight loss, they'll need an alternative—an effective weight-loss method. The reason is simple. Kids will continue to be unhappy with their weight and will want to change it. The method they need is the Naturally Thin Program, which focuses on eliminating famines. This is accomplished by always eating only high-class food in response to hunger signals, something from which kids and teens could benefit in many ways.

Eliminating famines entirely is difficult for most people because we are almost all accustomed to going hungry and eating lousy food, and it is deeply ingrained in us that going hungry is a good thing to do and junk food is unavoidable. Kids have to overcome these habits and prejudices regarding food and learn to eat whenever they are hungry. But just eating enough food won't necessarily break the Feast or Famine Cycle. Remember, two types of famines must be eliminated: quantity famines and quality famines.

KIDS AND EATING ON TIME

In order for our children to eliminate famines, we have to teach them to eat on time—right when they get hungry. The worst type of quantity famine is, of course, not eating at all when hunger signals occur. But if kids wait a half hour, an hour or even two after they first get hungry, they're "eating late," and this is a quantity famine, too. Anytime a person eats late, she is in a famine until she does eat and sets the adaptive responses of her body in motion.

If your child isn't especially "famine sensitive," then you may not see any changes in her/his eating or weight from going hungry or eating poor-quality food. This doesn't mean there is something wrong with her/his body; it just reflects a resistance to adaptive weight gain. In fact, most adolescents are quite resistant to significant weight gain even though dieting is a common practice, at least among girls, and most adolescents go hungry and eat junk food sometime every day. It may not be as critical for kids like this to be concerned about famines as those who are more famine sensitive, but they need to understand these principles anyway. Usually famine sensitivity increases with age.

Quantity famines seem to be just about as common as quality famines among adolescents. Kids skip breakfast (no time) and forget to pack their lunches (no foresight). At school, they borrow 50 cents and buy a bag of chips and share a Coke with a friend (no conscience). Girls may skip breakfast on purpose and pack an apple for lunch (no sense). Many skip lunch altogether. (They wonder why they are faint during gym class.) Young girls often see not eating as cool, while most boys eat plenty of lunch at school, since they are famished whether they ate breakfast or not. The girls are famished, too, but often deny it.

There's just one simple problem here: kids don't realize what they are doing to their bodies by their careless eating habits. Those who are not famine sensitive may not suffer weight gain as a consequence of eating like this, but some will slip into anorexia, and others will establish eating habits that may backfire later. Others will gradually gain and start dieting, setting themselves up for eating struggles that may last a lifetime. And those who are weight and diet conscious would be alarmed to learn what long-term effects all this food avoidance has on them. They must be told and reminded and helped to understand that eating enough good food when they are hungry is the only natural and healthful way to maintain an optimal weight.

But what if a kid doesn't want to be at an "optimal" weight? What if the kid is a wrestler and has to make weight (in order to compete), which is about eight pounds less than he "naturally" weighs? Or what if a girl doesn't feel thin enough at her natural weight because she is a bit thick and muscular like her parents, and her friends are all slim and angular? How are you going to get kids like this to stop going hungry?

Your power is certainly limited, but there's some simple information that you can share to help them—the facts about what they are doing to their bodies by undereating, and the physical reactions they are likely to get if they keep it up. If it doesn't shake them up right away, maybe it'll click in for them sometime down the road.

EARLY WARNING SIGNS

With all this teenage famining and dieting going on, it makes sense for any parent or adult who works with kids to be alert for precursors to the symptoms of eating disturbances. Usually months before an eating problem takes hold, signs of milder eating trouble can be recognized by a person who knows what they are and stays vigilant. These symptoms are associated with the Feast or Famine Cycle and include immoderate eating, heightened hunger, preoccupation with food and eating, cravings for sweets and fatty foods, signs of low metabolic rate (cold hands and feet, easily chilled, dry skin and hair). If a parent or other concerned person observes these symptoms, the cause must be explored, and if undereating is involved, the child needs to be educated about the Cycle and how she can get off it before she ends up in food jail.

FAMINE-SENSITIVITY TRAINING

There's a range of famine sensitivity in kids, just as there is in adults. Some kids just can't go hungry the same way others can without experiencing Cycle symptoms. They don't tolerate it. When they go hungry, their appetites soar and they almost immediately do make-up eating. Others who try dieting actually train their bodies to tolerate unsatisfied hunger. These kids are usually famine sensitive, too. Kids who have low famine sensitivity can eat or go hungry and it doesn't really affect them much. These kids, I have found, seem to be more vulnerable to anorexia than others.

It's probably a good idea to determine the famine sensitivity of your kids (see Chapter 2). If one of your children has a weight problem, it's obvious that she/he is more famine sensitive than most kids. Kids who are famine sensitive have to learn that their potential for weight gain in response to undereating and poor-quality diet is higher than other people's. They need to know that they don't have to eat less food than others their size to stay at a healthy weight, but they do have to eat better—always on time (when they first get hungry) and only high-quality food. They can't afford to go hungry or eat junk, and the sooner they learn it, the less pain and struggle they'll have.

EATING DURING SCHOOL

While we are teaching the ill effects of going hungry and eating nutrient-poor food, we had better consider accommodating our kids' fuel needs at school better. Most children I have interviewed, both lean and overweight, have confided their struggle with extreme hunger during the school day.

Tammy eats breakfast before 6:30 A.M. and doesn't get to the lunchroom before 12:30 P.M. (That's six hours! Twice as long as a kid should go without food.) Then she rushes through lunch because of play practice, which is scheduled during the last half of late lunch, and by the time school is out she usually feels light-headed and weak. Tammy was evaluated for low blood sugar (hypoglycemia) because of her symptoms, but there was no abnormality. She is simply not getting

*enough calories to keep up with her nutritional and energy
needs during the day because she can't—eating enough isn't
a priority at school. Besides, how much breakfast can a kid
eat to hold her for six hours?*

These kids complain of trouble concentrating the last two
classes before lunch. They become irritable. They say they don't
have any energy. And when they do eat, if they eat the school fare,
it's meager pickin's, and usually very high fat, which, of course,
they need because by then they are so extremely hungry they
could eat the erasers off their pencils.

We must do better. First, while we are teaching them in health
class how famines—going hungry and eating poor-quality food—
set the adaptive Cycles in motion, however subtly in the beginning, we've got to let kids eat sometime between breakfast and
lunch. And it would really help if we could make good food available at that morning break, say in vending machines in a canteen-
type room. Fresh fruit, yogurt, granola bars, milk, juices and even
sandwiches all fit nicely into vending machines. Teaching positive
eating and Cycle prevention has to be backed up by the environmental food supply we create for them at home and at school.

If this really isn't possible on a schoolwide basis, then at the
very least those kids who are famine sensitive (are overweight,
gain weight easily, have overweight parents) *must* be allowed to
eat when they need to between classes. Other kids will understand because they'll learn in health class why this is so important.

WHAT YOU CAN DO

Besides getting permission for individual children to snack during school hours, you can influence your child's school to offer
snack breaks to all students. Some parents simply approach the
principal with the suggestion of, and reasons for, mid-morning
snack breaks. (Snack foods are brought from home.) Others have
successfully worked with school nurses to make snacks part of the
morning schedule. Allow only Real Foods and make a snack suggestion list for parents along with a reminder of the importance of
feeding kids well before school, too.

HIGH-CALORIE, HIGH-QUALITY EATING

The term "high-calorie" usually strikes fear into the hearts of most diet-conscious people. But high-calorie eating is exactly what we need to teach our kids to do. They need quality calories, and plenty of them. No, there's no need to worry about overeating—it doesn't happen when people eat enough good food and never go hungry. And the good food part, well, we'll just have to keep working on that.

The caloric requirements of children and adolescents cover a very broad range, and are highly individualized depending on natural metabolic rate, activity level, weight, diet, growth activity and many other factors. Your child's caloric needs can be calculated by a nutritionist, but this is an estimate at best, and the caloric needs can change rather dramatically from day to day and month to month. A child's appetite should be the most reliable clue to determine how much food she needs, as long as the food is high quality only.

Calories are good. They are usable units of energy that make it possible for our bodies to function. But calories have a bad reputation in our country, and as a consequence, many people are trying to avoid calories by eating low-calorie and no-calorie foods. This is absurd. At best it keeps people who would otherwise enjoy eating freedom from enjoying it, and at worst it leads scores of innocent people into food jail. We must *tell* our kids that quality calories are good. We must help them become calorie and food friendly.

POSITIVE EATING AND CYCLE PREVENTION

It's a lot easier to keep kids off the Feast or Famine Cycle than it is to rescue them from it once they are ensnared. And the only way, really, to accomplish this is to warn them of the potential effects of going hungry and hope they take the message seriously. Some schools sponsor kids who have had eating disorders to talk with students and explain what happened to them. This can be a help if the visiting person has some insight about the role that dieting played in the development of her eating troubles. And most do. Some lace their stories with their emotional struggles, but almost all see dieting as at least the starting point. This is invaluable because kids tend to take peers' experiences more seriously than adults'. Besides personal pain, there's nothing like a person who has suffered from an affliction to impress kids and prove to them the reality of a dangerous path.

There are a few simple tips you can share to help your kids stay Cycle-free. They'll need to be reminded, probably many times, before these aids become habits. Write them down and post them on the refrigerator.

1. Never leave home without eating breakfast.
2. Take portable food with you wherever you go, especially if good food won't be available.
3. Always carry money with you to buy food.
4. Plan to eat somewhere about every three or four hours wherever you go.
5. Don't let other kids' eating habits interfere with your choices.
6. Make the best food choices you can in less than ideal situations.
7. Remind yourself that your body is capable of regulating your best weight if you keep eating enough good food whenever you're hungry.
8. Never, ever go hungry if you can help it.

These are good guidelines to follow yourself!

BODY ESTEEM

Body esteem is the sense of security and value that people have in their physical selves. Just as self-esteem is partly a function of the mirroring that we receive from people around us, body esteem can be influenced by people who are close to us—for better or worse. All children, and especially teenagers, need to be affirmed by others for being who they are—personally and also physically. The kind of affirmation that is most meaningful to kids is the free kind—support that they don't have to earn by working or performing. Kids all need to know that they are accepted and loved simply because they are, and they tend to thrive when they have this kind of security.

I remember once being bowled over by a situation that demonstrated the power of these principles. Hired to care for the children in a large family while the parents went on a trip, I can vividly recall being introduced to each family member, one by one, by a very proud mother who obviously took much delight in her handsome brood. And indeed, they were all exceptionally good looking. Not only that—they were obviously confident and very well adjusted kids. But one child was missing, and the mother explained that this teenage girl would join us shortly.

When this tardy family member arrived, I was quite startled. She smiled broadly as she extended her hand to me, obviously full of confidence like her siblings. But the thing that made her so unique was this: She was very homely. She had acne, her hair was dull and thin, her teeth were crooked, and she wore thick glasses that made her eyes look even smaller than they were. She had none of the classic features that her brothers and sisters shared in abundance. And she seemed absolutely oblivious to it. She was an ugly duckling surrounded by swans who really thought she was just as beautiful as the swans.

Do you know why? Her parents *told* her she was beautiful, in a hundred ways at least a thousand times during her life. Her parents believed, because she was theirs, that she *was* beautiful. She had been successfully indoctrinated by them to feel good about her physical self, to feel secure and attractive. And guess what? She eventually met and married a man who was very attractive, both inside and out, and they are living as happily ever after as anyone I know.

Everyone knows someone who has just the opposite profile: She feels ugly, fat and unattractive although she really is slim and beautiful. And it seems as if no amount of affirmation can change her attitude. She has been indoctrinated—especially by the culture, by her sensitive teenage perspective, perhaps by a cruel boyfriend or inattentive parents—with a poor body image. Is she hopeless? Is it too late for her to learn to appreciate and enjoy her physical self? Do body images get "locked in"? No, no, and sometimes.

Body image isn't a static thing. Many insecure teens, who once adamantly rejected their own bodies, grow through that painful stage into a more peaceful acceptance of their physical selves in their twenties. But when pregnancy temporarily ruins that peace for women not already caught in food jail, and dieting becomes a way of life, positive body image is likely to become an endangered asset.

HELPING KIDS LIKE THEIR BODIES

How can a parent or other person in a kid's life help build body esteem? Obviously things you say to your kids about their bodies can have a big impact, one way or another. Messages must be sincere, so don't make up things that you don't really believe. Focus on the kid's physical attributes that are strongest. This won't be hard with a kid who is naturally well proportioned and good looking, but every kid, even the plainest one, has some features worth reminding her about.

For instance, who can complain about a child's smile? OK, I know, teens rarely smile, but you can mention how wonderful her smile is in the class picture, and when she does smile, say you notice what a great smile she has. It may seem silly to you, but it can make a significant difference to a struggling teenager.

If she has thick, shiny hair, talk about that now and then. Notice it, mention it to her. If he has big shoulders (never mind that they're covered with acne), tell him you can see how big they are. If her ears are elegant, or her nose is classic, or his hands are huge, or her feet are shapely, or his legs are muscular, or her skin is milky, then *say* so. Don't just let the thought cross your mind or share the information with your sister: *Tell the kid.* Otherwise, they're more likely to dwell nonstop on what's wrong with their bodies and how they look, at least during their teens.

Kids have natural physical abilities to bring attention to as well. Some are lightning-fast runners. Others stand out at skating or batting or shooting hoops. Some are natural-born dancers and others do gymnastics with ease. Kids can be great bike riders or super trike riders or excellent floaters in the pool. Parents and other adults can make much of the most ordinary kid activities by noticing and talking about them. Watch for the areas where your kid is really enjoying her/his body, whatever her/his age, and then tell the kid that you enjoy watching her/him do physical things. This helps a kid appreciate what her body can do, her physical assets. It can also help de-emphasize appearance and thinness as the only important physical traits.

It's remarkable how many parents of young women with eating troubles routinely made disparaging comments about overweight people in their presence for years before their daughters' dieting and eating problems began. Undoubtedly, the things you say about other people's bodies around your kids send potent messages to them. Some messages kids pick up from these comments are:

I won't love or respect you if you ever get fat.
There is no excuse for people who gain extra weight—they simply don't make enough of an effort to avoid food.
Fat people are disgusting.
Fat people deserve to be mocked and ridiculed.
We are better than people who are more overweight than we.
Fat people aren't as valuable or worthwhile as thin people.

Different messages can be sent, but only if they reflect disparate attitudes. Here are a few:

Overweight people are handicapped, in a way.
People who are fat are trapped.
It would be very difficult to live as a fat person in our culture.
It isn't right to reject fat people just because they are overweight. In fact, it's prejudice.
It is nearly impossible for overweight people to get thin permanently.
Overweight people don't understand the role that dieting plays in causing their weight problem.
We all have struggles, and overweight people have the type of struggle that happens to show.

HOW PEOPLE SHOULD LOOK

Where do kids get their standards for looks? From the culture, of course, but parents can either reinforce the unhealthy and unrealistic messages of the culture or they can refute them. Kids are always listening for cues from the adults in their world. What standards are you holding up to kids? How can you reinforce more healthy and realistic body-image standards for the kids in your life?

With tears welling up in her eyes, Marion recalled a comment her dad had made when she tried on her first prom dress for him. Looking up briefly from his newspaper, he said

*matter-of-factly, "It makes you look chunky." And to Marion's
mother: "Don't you think the dress makes her look chunky?"
Marion had spent hours choosing the dress with her mother.
She was very excited about it and about going to the prom,
and she was devastated by her father's reaction to her appearance in this dress.*

*To tell the truth, Marion was chunky. She was built just like
her chunky father. There was no way to make her look tall
and svelte in a dress, or with diet and exercise. Marion was
short and thick, and it was genetic. Her dad didn't seem to
get it. But Marion got the message he sent: Your body isn't OK.
Tall and thin is the OK look. You have to be thinner to look attractive. That message sent Marion off on two years of
FeaFam Cycling.*

THE SETUP FOR EATING DISTURBANCES—
BODY-IMAGE TROUBLE

Is it an exaggeration that parents and other significant adults
have that much power over their kids' eating habits? No, it's no exaggeration. How kids see and feel about their bodies is almost always the single most important feature that separates kids who
develop eating problems from kids who don't. And parents and
other adults can profoundly affect kids' attitudes about their own
bodies.

If your comments can have such a powerful impact on kids'
body images, what about keeping silent? The things you don't say
about kids' bodies influence them, too. Most kids, and especially
most teenagers, need reassurance that their bodies are attractive,
that you are pleased with their physiques. And your reactions to
their requests for reassurance speak volumes.

Don't ridicule a kid who asks to be reassured about how she
looks. Take her seriously. If she looks fine, tell her plainly, many
times if necessary. If the kid doesn't look so great, tactfully suggest
some improvements. For example, "I like your hairstyle, but do
you think the nose ring seems to detract from it?" While kids are
developing their style they don't want you to lie to them about
what looks good and what doesn't, but there are sensitive ways to
get the truth across without shooting their fashion ideas down.

If a kid doesn't take your suggestions, don't be fooled into thinking that your input isn't valuable to her or him. The important thing is that you respond and pay attention without being overly critical. If she really does look disastrous, avoid overreacting, but don't lie just to keep the peace or to make her feel good. Even kids who are into kooky fashions can be supported in developing a healthy sense of their bodies by the adults around them. "That is really a wacky outfit, Jamie, but you sure put it together well. It's definitely a unique fashion statement!"

Of course, whether or not a kid looks to you for support regarding her appearance depends partly on your relationship. Kids who are more conforming, whose respect and admiration for their parents is closer to the surface, tend to rely more on them for opinions about how they look. But there's a twist here. Even rebellious kids who are at terrific odds with their parents can be extremely sensitive to remarks about how they look. So don't use this area of frustration—how a kid looks—to vent your anger at her about other things. It will only cause the rift between you to deepen and won't accomplish anything. And don't jeopardize a stable relationship by being insensitive about your kid's body-image concerns.

WHY ARE YOU LOOKING AT ME LIKE THAT?

Actions—and looks—speak louder than words. How you look at your kids is another powerful body-image message sender. If you really don't like how your kid looks physically, then you're probably going to let her know, whether or not you say so. You'll tell her in the expression on your face and through your body language. Well, what can you do about that? You can't just pretend she looks great when she looks horrible, can you? No, but that wouldn't work anyway because kids are really perceptive. What you can do is learn to be more tolerant of how kids look.

Brenda's acne and oily hair bothered her mother no end, and Brenda knew it. Her mother often sighed in frustration and held Brenda's stringy hair up in front of her eyes with a disgusted look on her face. She took Brenda shopping for special shampoos and pimple medications, but nothing helped much. Even with special shampoos, Brenda simply didn't wash her hair often enough, and her acne seemed to be unalterable. The seriousness of the problem became clear when Brenda accused her mother of hating her because of the "disgusted looks" she got.

Then Brenda's mom heard a counselor suggest that she try stepping back and looking at these problems as relatively unimportant in view of her daughter's whole life. She remembered that she had had these same troubles and somehow outgrew them without serious consequences. She realized that her relationship with her daughter was taking a beating because she wouldn't let these things go and allow her daughter to handle them. She decided to try looking at Brenda's stringy hair and pimply face with more humor, reminding herself that these troubles were sure to be temporary. And at the same time, she started making a real effort to send affirming messages to her daughter about her body, mainly by simply greeting her daughter with a smile.

These simple changes were almost like magic, and Brenda's mom enjoyed not only relief from her anxiety, but an improved relationship with Brenda as well. Oddly, after only a few weeks of these adjustments, Brenda started taking better care of her face and hair.

Reminding a kid about her physical qualities is one way to build a positive body image, but modeling body esteem sends a strong message, too. Kids pick up on our attitudes about our own bodies, whether or not we intend to share them. Little comments we make about how we think we look, the ways we use and enjoy and abuse our bodies, the comparisons we make between our bodies and others' all speak volumes to kids about our physical self-image. Adults who disparage their bodies, who complain that they aren't attractive, who focus on their physical liabilities are modeling poor body esteem to kids.

The best way to change this is to first develop a good body image yourself—no matter what you weigh, how tall you are, whether you are strong or weak, homely or beautiful. Positive body image is in the mind. Anybody can have it.

BODY-IMAGE MAKEOVER—REFRAMING YOUR CHILD'S PHYSICAL SELF-CONCEPT

What can a parent or other concerned person do for a kid who already has a negative body image? Are there ways to effectively encourage a better view of her physical self? Although there are certainly limits to how much a kid's body image can be affected from the outside, kids generally can be helped toward greater physical self-acceptance. I call this transformation a body-image makeover, and it is usually a long and gradual process.

Unlike a typical makeover where makeup and a new hairstyle change the actual appearance of a person, a body-image makeover happens on the inside of a person as well as on the outside. But some topical adjustments can help boost a kid's feelings about her body.

Outside changes that can help improve a kid's physical self-esteem include getting clothes that are flattering and big enough if the kid is, or thinks she is, overweight. Well-fitting and flattering clothes are extremely important to most kids, but especially those struggling with body-image troubles. Some basic grooming tactics can help add confidence, too—good haircuts, attractive jewelry, well-applied makeup and appealing fragrances.

Does this imply that you can purchase an improved body image? No, because there are issues here that go far deeper than the things money can change. A shaky body image may be helped a bit by these suggestions, but most body-image problems are resistant to topical solutions.

Body image is really an inside phenomenon—the subjective way an individual views her body and how she personally feels about her body, too. This subjectivity accounts for the blatant discrepancies between how kids actually look and their ideas of how they look. For instance, adolescent girls (and now preteens, too) often insist that they are fat when clearly they are not. Or they may think they are ugly when others see them as attractive. And sometimes they focus on one "terrible" flaw that becomes exaggerated in their minds and is a source of painful self-consciousness. Usually, others hardly notice this awful "defect."

What can we do to help kids through these painful body-image struggles? How can we help them develop more positive attitudes toward their bodies, flaws and all? Here are some suggestions:

Antidotes to Poor Body Image

1. Listen to kids when they complain about their bodies.

Irrational as they may sound, kids' concerns about their appearance are real and often upsetting to them. If they open up to you about this, it is very important that you allow them to share their concerns without denying the validity of their perspective. They may be irreverent: "I hate, absolutely loathe my legs! My ankles are like tree trunks and my thighs look like two Goodyear blimps! I wish I could cut them off!" Try not to react, but hear the strong feelings behind the expressions they use. Try to listen as a compassionate friend.

2. Never dismiss kids' worries or ridicule them for their body concerns.

"Sure, Tim, your nose is as big as a trumpet. You got it from your uncle Pinocchio," Tim's dad snickered when Tim complained about the increasing size of his nose. So Tim learned that he wasn't safe telling his dad about his body worries and wondered if there was something wrong with him because he worried about this stuff. And Tim's dad missed out on a chance to get closer to his son because he failed to take him seriously. Instead of making a joke because he couldn't see the problem Tim saw, Tim's dad could have reassured his son just by accepting his concern as legitimate.

3. Be truthful and sensitive when sharing your opinions about kids' appearances.

Don't lie to kids about their looks. They can detect insincerity and you'll lose your credibility. But don't be brutally honest, either. There are ways to tell hard truths gently. For instance, Chelsea is a cute preteen with a tire of fat padding around her middle. She picks out a bathing suit with ruffles around the middle, accentuating her apple shape. "Doesn't this look great?" she asks you. Here's what you say: "Chelsea, *you* look great, but the suit isn't the best style for you because it adds material to your middle and you already have enough material in the middle. Let's look for something in a solid with ruffles along the hips where you are smaller. You can use some extra material there."

4. Focus on positive aspects of a kid's appearance and body.

This point is redundant, but I can't emphasize it too much. Kids are sometimes extremely negative about their bodies at different times during their development. They need to be reminded of their bodies' good qualities to counterbalance the many things they'll find that disappoint them about the way they look. They can get this information only from outside, usually from the people they live with.

> *When Donna was sixteen she hated her body. Six feet tall and 135 pounds, she felt like a giant scarecrow without enough straw. She remembers agonizing over her frame with her mother, who always listened sympathetically and shared the struggle she had had as a very tall, thin teen. And Donna remembers something else her mother did. After she bemoaned her physical dimensions, Donna's mother would remind her what beautiful eyes she had and how she envied her for her thick, curly hair. And she'd talk about Donna's skill in volleyball, where her height was an important asset. Now twenty-six, Donna is a successful life insurance agent. She gives her mom credit for helping her to develop a strong self-image and an appreciation for her unique body.*

5. Remind kids that all bodies have imperfections.

It's best not to argue with a kid who insists that something about her body is totally gross. She's shooting from the hip—emotionally, that is. If you don't see this flaw the way the kid does, don't support her perception, but acknowledge that it's a real problem for her. After giving her plenty of time to say what she needs to say about it, you might add some perspective with a simple reminder: no body is perfect.

All bodies, however famous, have flaws or imperfections. Every beauty queen since time began has had "weak" features, but the smart ones just emphasize their strong points and come off looking perfect. Occasionally, an imperfection is used as a celebrity's signature, like the gap between Lauren Hutton's front teeth or the profile that could only belong to Barbra Streisand. Often physical faults can be minimized or modified, but they usually can't be changed completely. So everyone has to live with some problem area and shares the same challenge. This is offered to help your kid feel less alone in her struggle with physical flaws.

6. Share any body-image struggles you had as a kid in an empathetic way.

Kids often think their parents and other adults in their lives are far beyond the problems they face. They rarely understand that all adults have gone through many of the very same struggles. It can be a surprise and a relief to a kid who feels awkward about her body to learn that her mom or dad had some of the same thoughts and worries when they were her age.

> *"Mom, I've got to do something about my legs—they're huge compared to the rest of me," Carolyn complained to her mother. "I know gymnasts are supposed to be muscular, but the muscles on my legs are enormous! What can I do?"*
>
> *Her mother responded: "I absolutely hated my legs when I was your age. I was on the diving team and I had the biggest thighs on the team, including the boys'. It was maddening. I tried exercise and dieting, toning creams, the works. But nothing changed my legs. I had to learn to live with them, and they bothered me for years. So I know how you feel, and I wish I could help."*
>
> *"I didn't know you hated your legs! I mean, I wish I could trade with someone—anyone. Can you relate to this? I guess you can." Carolyn went on complaining, but her mom detected a slight lift in her voice.*

7. Remember that body image is subjective and slow to change.

Always bear in mind that people in general, and sometimes kids, too, are quite subjective about how they see their own physical selves. The unrealistic beliefs that people develop about their bodies are called distorted body image. Usually associated with eating disorders, body-image distortions can occur in anyone, and often do in teens. When these mental distortions are benign, kids just suffer some extra anxiety. But when body-image distortion is most malevolent, it involves the perception of overweight and leads its victims into food jail.

It's possible to wear down a misbelief that a kid holds about her body, but it takes time and many reminders of reality. Reassurance of physical attractiveness, desirability, proportion and normalcy may be rebuffed and received at the same time. But over time, kids usually recover more realistic perceptions of their bodies.

8. If a kid has a seriously distorted body image, see a counselor or therapist.

Kids who insist that there is something seriously wrong with their bodies or how they look, when there is not, should be seen by professionals. Strong delusions can reflect other problems that parents or unqualified adults can't assess. Sometimes this is a signal for help in a kid who doesn't know how to ask for it. Whatever these delusions might mean, don't ignore them.

"THE THIN IDEAL" AND POOR SELF-IMAGE

Just when kids are beginning to deal with who they are and what they're supposed to do with their lives, around age twelve, along comes *Teen Magazine* with its "Whatever Else You Are, You Must Be Extremely Thin to Be OK" message. Now by age twelve, the vast majority of kids are pretty skinny. It's the age of skinny, in fact. The ones who aren't skinny are likely to be getting into food jail already.

Then, wham! Between twelve and sixteen most girls pad up under the influence of hormones. Thinness and social acceptance become inseparable traits just when bodies are programmed to add fat. It's a setup for a terrific assault on the self-esteem of many—girls especially—an assault that all too often translates into eating disturbances. If food jail were a trap set to ensnare the most kids at the most vulnerable time of their lives, it couldn't be done more effectively than by the system we have now.

Self-esteem and thinness are unfortunately overlinked during the teen years. We've talked about boosting kids' body image to make them more resistant to the "Thinness Is Everything" message. But kids who have stronger self-esteem seem to be more resilient, too.

Insecurity and shaky self-esteem—rampant in young teens—leave kids more vulnerable to a whole host of self-destructive behaviors. Food jail usually doesn't rank with alcohol, drug use and sexual activity for destructive properties, but it should. Willful undereating is not only physically harmful, but it seriously adds to the emotional turmoil of the age as well. Blood-sugar and mood swings go together. Undersatisfied hunger and lethargy fit, too. Going hungry usually brings even more irritability to already crabby teens.

Building kids' self-esteem is the central topic of many books, and any parents or concerned adults would do well to educate themselves on the topic. Broadly speaking, kids' self-esteem develops well when their most basic needs are consistently met—in an atmosphere of love and respect. After food, clothing, shelter and safety, kids' most basic needs include the need for discipline (teaching and consequences) and the need for healthy relationships. Kids need to know they are loved and accepted without strings—without having to earn it. And they need to know that they're not alone—that they won't be abandoned no matter what. Kids who have these needs met usually have better self-esteem and personal security than those who don't.

No parent can meet her kids' needs perfectly, and even if she did, kids would still struggle with self-esteem, more or less. So if your kid has poor self-esteem, don't beat yourself up. Learn how to support her in developing a better one, with counseling if necessary. Read those books, join a parents' support group. It's one more important antidote to food jail, and other adolescent pitfalls as well.

• REAL FOODS

Breads, Grains, Cereals

All breads, whole-grain preferred
Bagels, English muffins, pretzels, whole-grain crackers
All unsweetened cold or hot cereals, preferably whole-grain
Pasta, all types
Rice, including brown, wild and white (not fried)
Sandwiches made with Real Food fillings
Dumplings, stuffing*
Muffins, whole-grain preferred

Legumes, Nuts and Seeds

Seeds of all types*
Nuts of all kinds*
Peanut butter*
Almond butter, other nut/seed spreads*
Beans

Fruits and Vegetables

All fruits, fresh preferred, canned, stewed
All vegetables, fresh and lightly cooked preferred, canned, frozen
Vegetable-based dishes, like Oriental stir-fry, vegetable casseroles, vegetables with
    rice
Fruit jams and jellies
Juices, 100 percent unsweetened fruit or vegetable juice
Salads made from Real Foods
Soups, broth-based preferred

Dairy and Eggs

Milk, low-fat or nonfat
Cheese*
Cottage cheese, low-fat or nonfat
Yogurt, low-fat or nonfat, preferably sugar-free or sweetened with fruit juice (to avoid
        the empty calories of refined sugar)
Cream, as a flavoring*
Sour cream, low-fat or nonfat
Milk/cream-based soups*
Eggs

Meat, Poultry, Seafood

Beef, lean cuts
Chicken, skinless, white meat preferred
Fish, all types
Turkey and other poultry, skinless, white meat preferred
Hamburger, extra lean*
Pork, lean cuts
Shellfish
Soups, broth-based
Stews, fat-skimmed

Fats, Spreads

To optimize your diet, use high-fat types, like butter or peanut butter, sparingly and
earlier in the day, and buy fat-free or fat-reduced mayonnaise. Otherwise, anything used
on the teaspoon level is OK.

Condiments

Mustard, vinegar, relishes
Fresh or dried herbs and spices
Sugar, syrup
Ketchup, barbecue sauce, hot sauce, salsa
Steak sauce, Worcestershire sauce
Fruit dips*
Veggie dips*
Salad dressings*
Jelly, jams and preserves

Beverages

Unsweetened fruit juices
Vegetable juices
Sugar-free beverages—diet pop, powdered drinks
Coffee, regular or decaf
Tea, regular, decaf or herbal
Hot chocolate*

· BORDERLINE FOODS

Avoid these foods as much as possible and stay "fed up" on Real Foods! OK to eat in an emergency situation, but try to keep enough quality food with you to stay away from Borderlines. Always pick the best quality foods among poor quality choices.

Fried ANYTHING
"Munchies" like popcorn, chips, most crackers
Fast foods, except the lower-fat or "light" options
Sweet rolls, pastries, etc.
Bacon, sausage, processed meats (salami, bologna)
Waffles, restaurant pancakes
Pudding, custard, sweetened yogurt
Presweetened cereals and oatmeal
Punch, soft drinks, all sugar-based drinks
Casseroles with high fat content
Cream-based soups, stews
Lamb, spareribs
Frozen pot pies, regular frozen dinners
Pizza, especially with pepperoni, sausage, etc. (Homemade pizza with natural tomato
        sauce and low-fat mozzarella or ricotta cheese is OK.)

NOTE: IF THE INGREDIENTS ARE FROM THE REAL FOODS LIST, AND ARE LOW FAT OR LOW SUGAR IT'S OK.

*Indicates that this Real Food or beverage may have high fat content so check ingredients if you eat this frequently because substitutes can be made to improve the quality. Otherwise, these richer foods are to be eaten less often, say as a treat every few weeks rather than regularly. This is not because there is something inherently evil about fattier foods. It's because a high-quality diet is always lower in fat, with no more than 30 percent of the total calories coming from fat.

• PLEASURE FOODS

Unless you are immune to the effects of dessert indulgence, do not allow Pleasure Foods any kind of significant place in your diet. If cravings continue, signaling that you still need these treats, keep working on getting off the Cycle so you can be free of them. Once in a great while, like every three or four months in a very special situation, go ahead, just for the pleasure. If you're off the Cycle, it won't do much for you anyway.

Cakes, frosting
Chocolate
Candy bars, candy
Cookies and bars
Coffee cakes
Fudge
Betties, cobblers, strudel, etc.
Pies, pastries
Ice cream, sherbet, frozen yogurt
Sweet toppings, ice cream and dessert syrups

lifestyle of, 83–86, 90, 92
loss of control in, 63–64
low-fat type, 145–46
mind-controlled famines and,
    109–10
myths and false tenets of,
    95–102, 209–10
national obsession with, 15, 59,
    98–99
Naturally Thin Program vs.,
    109–20
overweight and, 22, 23, 25
"payoffs" from, 31, 62, 70, 83
preoccupation with, 85, 86
rebounding effect of, 64–65
reinforcements of, 62–63, 83
self-punishment and, 62–63
statistics on, 59, 60–61
stopping cycle of, 86–87, 94–107
"success" with, 86
withdrawal from, 90–94
in your future, 164–65
yo-yo, 69, 235
see also compulsive undereating
diet or anti-eating cults, 12
diet prescriptions, 102–7
Dr. Atkins' Diet Revolution
    (Atkins), 99

eating:
    adaptive make-up, 28, 67, 96
    body-controlled, 218–19
    obsession with, 15–31
eating-avoidance, *see* food-avoidance
eating disorders:
    acute and dangerous types of,
        235–37
    adaptation mechanisms as paral-
        lel to symptoms of, 10, 45–51
    anxiety and, 21, 28, 93–94, 149–50
    appetites and, 44, 45, 46–47
    checklist for eating patterns in,
        34–35
    children and adolescents, *see*
        eating disorders in children

    and adolescents
chronic and stable types of,
    235–37
common denominator in, 22–23,
    30–31
concern for others with, *see* eat-
    ing disorders in other people
confusing symptoms of, 226–27
definitions of, 18, 30
dieting and undereating as set
    up for, 10, 22, 23, 25, 35–36,
    43–44, 56
empowerment over, 70, 221–24
failure of therapy in treatment
    of, 29, 30
famine factor role in, 32–55
fear of food and, 24, 51, 75,
    76–77, 218
Feast or Famine Cycle and, 56–77
food availability factors leading
    to, 52–54
food hunger vs. love hunger in,
    24–28
health issues in, 223, 235–37
liberation from, 69–70
loss of control of eating and, 21,
    27, 37, 46–47, 71, 81–82
psycho-emotional theories on,
    11, 18, 23, 24, 28–30, 160,
    205–7
recovery from, 77, 81–200
survival-instinct role in, 9, 10, 30,
    43–51
symptoms of, 10, 24, 33–36, 65,
    86, 233
types and descriptive labels of,
    19–31
understanding the basis of, 15–77
withdrawal symptoms in over-
    coming of, 91–94, 126
see also specific disorders
eating disorders in children and
    adolescents, 250–75
body-controlled eating and,
    218–19

---

healthy, normal eating (cont.)
    withdrawal symptoms and, 91–94
How to Become Naturally Thin by Eating More (Antonello), 11
hunger:
    anorexia and, 90
    appetite control mechanism and, 46–47
    emotions, stress and, 149–50
    food and love in, 24–28
    ignoring of, 24, 139
    medicating of, 140
    satisfaction of, 96–98, 99, 102–3
    signals of, 135, 136–37, 138, 142–43, 149
    survival instinct's effect on, 44

intervention, 232, 235–36

ketones, 90
liquid diets, 62, 211
loss of appetite, stress and, 25

men and boys, athletics and, 61
metabolic rate, 43, 45, 46, 53, 121, 122
mirrors, 156–57
mood elevators, biochemical, 90

"naturally thin," 51–52, 61, 100, 123, 144
Naturally Thin Program, 94–108, 115, 200, 203–24
    body-controlled eating in, 109–15, 117–19
    case histories in, 167–200
    doctrines of, 94–102
    helping others in, 203–75
    new body image in, 147–66
    period of adjustment to, 116, 126–31
    prescriptions of, 102–8
    recovery and, 122–34
    support resources for, 107–8
    traditional dieting vs., 109–46

obesity, see overweight
OPIOOM (other peoples inferred opinions of me) addiction, 165–66
Overeaters Anonymous (OA), 25, 26, 67–68, 178, 185, 199–200
overeating, see compulsive overeating; overweight
overweight:
    adaptive fat storage and, 45–51
    bias in scientific research on, 36, 203–9
    cultural prejudices, beliefs and attitudes on, 18, 24, 83–84, 205
    diet industry's promotion of, 51, 68–69
    dieting as start of, 9, 10, 22, 23, 25, 207–9
    erroneous beliefs and, 17, 18, 24, 28
    fear of food and, 10, 17
    food-avoidance and fear of, 36–37
    genetic predisposition for, 53–54
    lack of exercise and, 17, 18, 49, 101
    overeating as symptom vs. cause of, 28–30
    paradox of undereating and, 25
    professional treatment of, 18–19, 29, 30, 203–4, 207, 210–11
    resistance to, 51–52
    self-punishment and guilt of, 62–63, 85
    undereating in relation to, 10

pleasure food, 280
presenting food, 111
primary dependence, 228, 229

rebounding dieter, 64–66, 76
recovery, 81–200
    doctrines for, 94–102
    empowerment for, 69–70, 77, 221–24
    evaded issues surfacing in, 92–93
    exercise and, 105–6